HYPERTHERMIA

ADVANCES IN EXPERIMENTAL MEDICINE AND BIOLOGY

HYPERTHERMIA

Edited by
Haim I. Bicher
Western Tumor Medical Group
Van Nuys, California

and
Duane F. Bruley
Louisiana Technical University
Ruston, Louisiana

PLENUM PRESS • NEW YORK AND LONDON

Library of Congress Cataloging in Publication Data

North American Hyperthermia Group. Meeting (1st: 1981: Detroit, Mich.)
  Hyperthermia.

(Advances in experimental medicine and biology; v. 157)
  "Proceedings of the First Annual Meeting of the North American Hyperthermia
Group (NAHG), held August 23–25, 1981, in Detroit, Michigan"—P.
  Includes bibliographical references and index.
  1. Thermotherapy—Congresses. 2. Cancer—Treatment—Congresses. I. Bicher,
Haim I. II. Bruley, Duane F. III. Title. IV. Series. [DNLM: 1. Fever therapy—Con-
gresses. 2. Neoplasms—Therapy—Congresses. W1 AD559 v.157/QZ 266 H997 1981]
RC271.T5N67 1981   616.99′0632   82-18047
ISBN 0-306-41172-5

Proceedings of the First Annual Meeting of the North American
Hyperthermia Group (NAHG), held August 23–25, 1981, in Detroit, Michigan

©1982 Plenum Press, New York
A Division of Plenum Publishing Corporation
233 Spring Street, New York, N.Y. 10013

Printed in the United States of America

Meeting: Organizing Committee

Chairman: Haim I. Bicher M. D.

D. Leeper, Ph.D.
K. Storm, M. D.
C. W. Song, Ph.D.
D. F. Bruley, Ph.D.

NAHG Organizing Committee

J. S. Bedford
H. I. Bicher
P. M. Corry
W. C. Dewey
E. W. Gerner
L. E. Gerweck
E. W. Hahn
G. M. Hahn
G. M. Hetzel
N. B. Hornback

D. B. Leeper
J. R. McLaren
G. H. Nussbaum
J. R. Oleson
H. P. Plenk
T. S. Sandhu
C. W. Song
J. R. Stewart
F. K. Storm

PREFACE

Hyperthermia is rapidly becoming the fourth modality of cancer treatment, at least a useful adjuvant to radiation therapy, chemotherapy or surgery; at best, a new therapeutic form that, properly used, may open new horizons in the fight against this dreadful disease.

The staging is still primitive. The devices used are after laboratory improvisations, and lack the precision and definition of treatment fields that will allow mass use of the modality. Clinical practices are limited to the procedural evaluations of a few pioneer groups, and basic understanding of its mechanism of action, although progressing by leaps and bounds, is still short of perfection.

The challenge and the promise are there, and because of this, engineers, physicists, biologists, physiologists and clinicians from different specialties have a basic need for interaction, both in terms of exchange of scientific information and peer review of results and clinical trials. To satisfy this need, to act as a clearinghouse of knowledge and a forum for discussion, the North American Hyperthermia Group (NAHG) has been formed. The meeting in Detroit in August 1981 represents the first gathering of the group, to be followed by a second in Salt Lake City in April 1982.

The Detroit meeting was mostly devoted to the physiology and clinical problems associated with Hyperthermia, although physics and basic thermobiology were also discussed. 75 scientists attended the meeting and 30 papers were presented. A selection of these papers represents this volume, offered more as a statement of problems than a final solution to them.

We hope that many meetings will follow, that Hyperthermia will become a useful clinical modality, and that NAHG, perhaps in a more organized fashion, will play the future role that its founders envisaged.

Haim I. Bicher
Duane F. Bruley
June, 1982

CONTENTS

IDENTIFICATION OF VIABLE REGIONS IN "IN VITRO" SPHEROIDAL TUMORS:

A MATHEMATICAL INVESTIGATION

Nathan A. Busch, Duane F. Bruley, and Haim I. Bicher

Biomedical Engineering Department, Louisiana Tech
University, Ruston, Louisiana, 71270 and Western Tumor
Medical Group and Valley Cancer Institute, 5522 Sepulveda
Van Nuys, California, 91411

ABSTRACT

In the treatment of solid tumors by hyperthermia, a major
question is how to obtain an a priori knowledge of which tumors can
be effectively treated with this modality. The key question is;
given a solid tumor, what parameters in the various regions of the
tumor, need to be measured so that a tumor-tissue model can provide
a meaningful real time simulation of the hyperthermic treatment.
This paper addresses the former question as a mathematical investigation, and the latter as a consequence of the former.

INTRODUCTION

Microspheriods of tumor cells have proven useful as in vitro
tumor models. These spheroids are thought to have central cells
which suffer from nutritional stresses causing them to have a
chronically hypoxic, radioresistant fraction of cells. In this study,
direct microphysiological determination of the oxygen tension in
spheriods has been made. Since it is known that the sensitivity of
the tumor cells to radiation and hyperthermia is related to the
oxygen level in the environment, the potential success of combined
hyperthermia-radiation treatment will be influenced by the
distribution of oxygen in the tumors (1). These oxygen profiles
when accurately predicted by a mathematical model of the system
yield valuable information for the development of an understanding
as to what characteristics an in vivo tumor must have to be successfully treated by hyperthermia. The information provided by this
study can be used in mathematical models of tumor hyperthermia (3).

1

Oxygen profiles in 300 micron spheroids were averaged to give a representative profile from which to work (2). A mathematical model describing the diffusion and metabolism of oxygen in the spheriod was developed. The oxygen diffusion equation was written for the bath, in which no metabolism occurred. The equations, which are dependent only on radial position, were solved to yield the radially dependent oxygen tensions in both the bath and spheroid. The profiles were then fit to the statistically representative profile to determine important model parameters for further utilization.

METHODOLOGY

The cell line used for the spheroid tumor studies were Chinese hamster lung fibroblasts (V79) maintained in Eagle's Basal Medium supplemented with 15% fetal calf serum in spinner flasks.

The experimental oxygen level data used for mathematical comparison were determined using polarographic techniques with gold in glass ultramicroelectrodes of tip diameter 1 to 5 microns (4). The electrodes were coated with oxygen permeable membranes of Formvar and Rhoples. The reference electrode was a Ag/AgCl wire of 1 mm. diameter.

Mathematical equations describing the diffusion and metabolism of oxygen in a spherical tumor were derived from basic principles. The equations provide for changing the metabolic rate term depending upon where in the tumor the solution is being obtained. This feature allows for the analysis of regional differences in oxygen consumption. The analysis indicates which regions contain cells that are viable, radiosensitive, and which regions contain cells that are not radio-sensitive. The cells which are radioresistive are those which can be effectively treated with chemotheraputic drugs to make them more radiosensitive.

The equation describing the diffusion and metabolism of oxygen in a spherical tumor is

$$\frac{d^2\psi_t}{d\xi^2} + \frac{2}{\xi}\frac{d\psi_t}{d\xi} = R_m$$

$$R_m = \frac{r_t^2 Q_{O_2,1}}{P_{O_2,b}(\infty)\, D_{O_2,t} S_{O_2,t}} \qquad \text{when } p_1^* < \psi_t \; p_o^*$$

$$\frac{r_t^2 Q_{O_2,2} \Psi_t}{D_{O_2,t} S_{O_2,t}}$$

when $p_2^* < \Psi_t < p_1^*$

$$\frac{r^2 Q_{O_2,3} \Psi_t}{D_{O_2,t} S_{O_2,t} (K_{M,O_2} + P_{O_2,t}(\infty) \Psi_t)}$$

when $p_3^* < \Psi_t \ p_2^*$

where

$$p_o^* = P_{O_2,b} \ / \ P_{O_2,b}(\infty) = 1.0$$

$$p_1^* = P_{O_2,b}(r_1) \ / \ P_{O_2,b}(\infty)$$

$$p_2^* = P_{O_2,b}(r_2) \ / \ P_{O_2,b}(\infty)$$

$$p_3^* = P_{O_2,b}(r_3) \ / \ P_{O_2,b}(\infty)$$

$$\Psi_t = P_{O_2,t}(r) \ / \ P_{O_2,b}(\infty)$$

$$\xi = r \ / \ r_t$$

The equation for the oxygen profile utilizes three types of consumption in the tumor. Each type of consumption occurs within a definite range of oxygen tension levels. The regional boundaries and kinetic parameters are determined by fitting computed oxygen profiles to the experimental profiles.

The equation for the diffusion of oxygen in the medium outside the tumor is

$$\frac{d^2 \Psi_b}{d\xi} + \frac{2}{\xi} \frac{d\Psi_b}{d\xi} = 0$$

where

$$\Psi_b = P_{O_2,b}(r) \ / \ P_{O_2,b}(\infty)$$

These equations were solved using an Adams Moulton Bashforth technique. The unknowns in the system were determined by the Newton-Rapheson technique. The constraint equations for the Newton-Rapheson technique are:

$$\Psi_b(1.06) = \Psi_{b,exp}(1.06)$$

$$\Psi_t(1.00) = \Psi_{t,exp}(1.00)$$

$$\Psi_t(\xi : \Psi_{t,exp} = p_3^*) = p_3^*$$

The first constraint equation states that the oxygen tension
in the bath in the region of the tumor is lower than the tension in
the bath far away from the tumor. The thickness of this boundary
is 1.06 times the radius of the tumor (for the set of tumors used
in this study). The second equation requires that the measured
and computed oxygen tension at the surface of the tumor be the same.
The third equation states that the computed and measured oxygen
tension be the same at the radial position where the consumption
rate term changes from first order to Michaelis-Menton.

There are four more constraints to be imposed on the system.
These are the boundary conditions. At the center of the tumor,
the oxygen tension gradient and level of oxygen tension are specified
to be the same as were experimentally measured. There are two
bath boundary conditions which must be specified. The two bath
boundary conditions were for the tumor-bath interface. The first
boundary condition required that the oxygen gradient for the bath
was proportional to the gradient for the tumor. The second condition
was that the bath and tumor oxygen tension at the interface were
the same.

The unknowns in the system are the tumor oxygen diffusivity-
solubility product, the first order reaction rate constant, and the
Michaelis-Menton reaction rate constant. Once the constants were
accurately determined, the simulation was again ran to compute the
oxygen tension profiles in the tumor. Plotting the computed, and
experimetal profile vs. radial position illustrates the agreement
between the two curves.

RESULTS AND ANALYSIS

The physical parameters used in the simulation are given in
Table 1. Included in this table are the numerically determined
values of the tumor oxygen diffusivity, (assuming a tumor oxygen
solubility) the first order kinetic constant and Michaelis-Menton
reaction rate constants. These parameters were determined by
matching the experimentally measured and computed oxygen profiles.
The computed and experimental oxygen profiles vs. radial position
are plotted in Figure 1.

The regions of different metabolism are separated by a sharp
dividing line at a depth of 40 microns, or at a radius of 110 microns.
This sharp division line suggests that the outer 40 microns of the
tumor contain viable cells which have an adequate oxygen supply to

TABLE 1

NOMENCLATURE:

$D_{0_2,t}$ Diffusivity of oxygen in the tumor, $cm^2/sec.$

$K_{M,0_2}$ Michaelis-Menton constant for oxygen in the tumor, mm Hg.

p_0^* Dimensionless oxygen partial pressure of the bath at infinity.

p_1^* Dimensionless oxygen partial pressure in the tumor at which the consumption rate changes from zeroth order to first order in oxygen.

p_2^* Dimensionless oxygen partial pressure in the tumor at which the consumption rate changes from first order to Michaelis-Menton kinetics.

p_3^* Dimensionless oxygen partial pressure in the tumor at which the consumption of oxygen ceases.

$P_{0_2,b}$ Oxygen partial pressure in the bath, mm Hg.

$P_{0_2,t}$ Oxygen partial pressure in the tumor, mm Hg.

$S_{0_2,b}$ Solubility of oxygen in the bath, $cm^3-0_2/(cm^3-$ tissue mm Hg).

$S_{0_2,t}$ Solubility of oxygen in the tumor, $cm^3-0_2/(cm^3-$ tissue mm Hg).

Ψ_b Dimensionless oxygen tension in the bath.

Ψ_t Dimensionless oxygen tension in the tumor.

ξ Dimensionless radial distance.

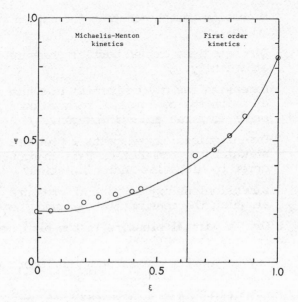

Figure 1.   Dimensionless oxygen tension (ξ) vs. dimensionless radial position (ξ).

make them radiosensitive. However, the inner 110 microns of tumor consists of cells which are not viable, and are radioresistive. This line of demarcation between the two zones of cells is determined by changing the oxygen tension at which the metabolism changes from first order to Michaelis-Menton kinetics until a good fit of the data is made. Of course, the values of the physical parameters are dependent upon the position of this line of demarcation, which complicates the problem of determining its location accurately (numerical trial and error calculations).

CONCLUSIONS

A mathematical model has been developed for diffusion and metabolism of oxygen in tumor spheroids. A numerical technique has been developed which calculates the values of the diffusion constants in the spheroid the first order and Michaelis-Menton kinetic constants, as well as the point of demarcation from first order to Michaelis-Menton reaction. This method yields values for the parameters which produce an accurate prediction of the oxygen profile behavior in in vitro spherical tumors.

This study calculates the oxygen tension distribution in spheroids. By using the different types of oxygen consumption to obtain a fit between experimentally measured and computed oxygen tension profiles, the different regions of cell viability may be correlated with their respective consumption rates.

REFERENCES

1. Bicher, H. I., F. W. Hetzel, T. S. Sandhu, S. Frinak, P. Vaupel, M. O'Hara, and T. O'Brien, "Effects of Hyperthermia on Normal and Tumor Microenvironment," Radiology, 137, 521-530, (1980).
2. Bicher, H. I. and P. Marvin, "Pharmacological Control of Local Oxygen Regulation Mechanisms in Brain Tissue," Stroke, Volume 7, 469-472, (1976).
3. Busch, N. A., D. F. Bruley, and H. I. Bicher, "Computer Modeling of Tumor Hyperthermia," this publication.
4. Kaufman, N., H. I. Bicher, F. W. Hetzel, and M. A. Brown, "A System for Determining the Pharmacology of Indirect Radiation Sensitizer Drugs on Multicellular Spheroids," Cancer Clinical Trials, Volume 4, 199-204, (1981).

HYPERTHERMIA FOR MALIGNANT DISEASE – A HISTORY OF MEDICINE NOTE –

THE WORK OF GEORGES LAKHOVSKY

Kevin Farrell, M.D.

Department of Surgery, West Virginia University School
of Medicine - Morgantown, West Virginia 26506

As hyperthermia is becoming more important in the treatment
of malignant disease, it is appropriate to bring attention to the
life and work of one of the pioneers in the field, Georges Lakhovsky,
who is today a forgotten man. Georges Lakhovsky was born in Illia,
Russia (near Minsk) in 1870. He studied engineering at Odessa and
came to France in 1894 where he studied physics at the University
of Paris. He remained in France, married, and became a naturalized
french citizen. During the first world war he was attached to the
French Army and devised an improved method of laying railroad tracks.
He elucidated a rule (The "Lakhovsky Rule") which was used in
predicting failure of railroad tracks. For this work he was awarded
a medal and given a commendation by the French government.

After the first world war he became interested in wireless
transmission. It was through this work that he became interested
in the Biologic Application of Radio Waves. Although he is not
generally given credit for it, he was the first person to design
and build what is today called a "Short Wave Diathermy" machine.
His first experiments with this machine in the production of
artificial fever were carried out in 1923, In conjunction with
french physicians he used this machine and subsequent modifications
of it to treat patients with malignant tumors. This work was done
at the Hospital de la Salpetriere (with Professor Gosset) and at
the Hospital Saint-Louis (with Dr. Louste). These are two well-
known hospitals in Paris. The first patient was treated at the
Hospital de la Salpetriere in 1924. The frequencies that Lakhovsky
used were from 0.75 megahertz to 3000 megahertz. This is within
the range that is being used today in clinical hyperthermia. In
1931 he began using a machine that emitted radio waves of multiple
different wavelengths.

9

Although a controversial figure in his time, he did have some success with his treatments. He presented reports of his work at the Pasteur Institute and French Academy of Sciences. His work was cited in an english language book on the biologic effects of radiation (1) and a book was written about his life and work (2).

As a Jew who had written an anti-fascist book, he fled France in 1940 and came to New York City where he died in 1942. I believe he was the first person to use radio frequency electromagnetic radiation in the treatment of human tumors. It is hoped that he will no longer remain a forgotten man.

1. Cited in the section by G. Murray McKinly in Biological Effects of Radiation. Edited by Duggar, Published in 1936.
2. La Vie Et Les Ondes, L'Oeuvre De Georges Lakhovsky by Michel Adam and Armand Givelet, Etienne Chiron, Paris, 1936.

An abreviated bibliography of Georges Lakhovsky is listed below. (A more extensive bibliography can be obtained from the author of this paper.)

1. Comptes Rendus Des Seances De L'Academie Des Sciences - Volume L84, p. 907 (April 4, 1927), Volume L86, p. 1019 (April 11, 1928), Volume 188 pp. 657, 659 (Feb. 25, 1929), Volume 188 pp. 1069, 1071 (April 15, 1929), Volume 192 p. 1048 (May 26, 1931)
2. Revue Generale Des Sciences - March 11, 1927, April 30, 1928, Oct. 15, 1928, June 15, 1927, June 30, 1928, July 15, 1928, Dec. 15, 1928, April 30, 1934.
3. La Revue Scientifique - May 14, 1927, May 25, 1931, Aug. 11, 1934.
4. La Revue Medicale Francaise - April 1, 1931, May 1, 1931.
5. Lhospital - December, 1932.
6. Journal De Medecine De Paris - Dec. 25, 1930.
7. La Gazette Des Hospitaux - May 4, 1929, May 16, 1934.
8. Journal De Medecine (Lyon) - April 5, 1933, April 5, 1934.
9. Journal De Physiologie Et De Pathologie Generale - March, 1935.
10. Paris Medical - May 18, 1935.
11. Journal Des Sciences Medicales De Lille - Sept. 3, 1933.

SEQUENTIAL REGIONAL HYPERTHERMIA: A POSSIBLE ANSWER

FOR THE TREATMENT OF CANCER

John M. Rude' and Howard L. Mark

CompuMed, Inc., Los Angeles, California

HYPERTHERMIA AND METASTATIC CANCER

Abstract

A therapeutic rationale for the treatment of metastatic cancer
is presented which incorporates the use of deep regional hyperthermia of major body areas such as the thorax and abdomen. These
body areas would be treated sequentially with the goal of eliminating
the problems inherent to whole-body hyperthermia. To achieve this
goal, a tri-modality approach is considered which combines regional
deep heating with regional X-ray therapy and with drug therapy
using agents which are heat as well as radiation hypoxic cell
sensitizers (Nitroimidazoles or glucose analogues). The rationale
for such an approach is well founded at the basic research level.
The benefit of the tri-modality approach is that therapeutic levels
of drug, X-rays and heat can be reduced significantly and hopefully
be non-toxic.

A Possible Answer for the Treatment of Metastatic Cancer

This paper presents a rationale for treating deep-seated
metastatic cancer with hyperthermia in combination with radiation
and drugs. The drugs to be discussed are both heat and radiation
cell sensitizers and in addition act preferentially on tumor cells
(as opposed to conventional chemotherapeutic drugs). Our approach
is based on the concept of sequential regional hyperthermia of large
body regions (e.g. thorax, abdomen) and is made feasible by recent
technological advances which have led to regional deep-heating
machines such as the Magnetrode and the BSD phased annular array.
The ultimate success of these machines strictly from an engineering

11

viewpoint will be proven with time. One important characteristic
of these machines is their ability to heat deep-seated tumors to
therapeutic temperatures (42-44C) within 10-15 minutes. This
contrasts with the characteristic long (2-3 hr.) heat-up times
associated with whole-body hyperthermia.

While hyperthermia alone can lead to palliative effects and
to regression of tumors, its ultimate success in the cure of tumors
appears to depend on combined modality therapy. In combination with
X-ray therapy, hyperthermia is proving to be a very effective local
cancer therapy modality (1,3,7,8,9,13). How then to effectively
combine X-rays with hyperthermia in the treatment of large body
regions such as the abdomen and thorax.

Radiation therapy dictates that the abdominal as well as
thoracic regions be limited to a maximum X-ray dose of approximately
2000 rads delivered in daily fractions of approximately 175 r. This
maximum total dose of X-rays is limited by lung toxicity in the
thorax and by kidney toxicity in the abdomen. Together however,
the thorax and abdomen account for approximately 80% of the bone
marrow of the whole body, and whole body irradiation is limited by
bone marrow toxicity. Therefore, in order to irradiate both the
abdomen and thorax with 2000 r, a recovery period for bone marrow
(6-8 weeks) would be required in between treatment of the 2 body
regions.

The radiation protective drug, WR-2721, which is currently
undergoing Phase I clinical trials (10), potentially could play an
important role in sequential regional therapy involving hyperthermia
and X-rays. WR-2721 protects most normal tissues (not brain or
spinal cord), but not tumors from x-irradiation (see Table 1 &2)
(24). Organs and tissues which are critical with respect to radiation toxicity are protected (in animals) by factors of 1.5 - 3.0
by WR-2721 (see Table 1). The effect which WR-2721 theoretically
(predicted from animal data) would have in the clinic on the
maximum X-ray dose tolerable to thorax* and abdomen as well as on
the bone marrow recovery time is illustrated in Table 3.

Preliminary experiments (J. Yuhas, Personal communication)
have shown that in mice, hyperthermia does not alter the pharmacology of WR-2721: namely that normal tissues still absorb the
drug while tumors do not. However, as Yuhas (23) has pointed out,
if hyperthermia is administered after WR-2721 and X-rays, then
independently of any interaction between WR-2721 and hyperthermia,
WR-2721 should prevent synergistic interactions of radiation and
hyperthermia in normal tissues merely by reducing the radiation-
injury component.

*Recent data (J. Yuhas, personal communication) confirm a protect-
ion factor for lung of 1.8-2.0.

TABLE 1

SUMMARY OF NORMAL TISSUE RESPONSIVENESS TO
PROTECTION BY WR-2721[a]

Tissues Which Are Protected	Tissues Which Are Not Protected
1. Bone marrow (2.4-3.0)[b]	1. Brain
2. Immune system (1.8-3.4)	2. Spinal cord
3. Skin (2.0-2.4)	
4. Small intestine (1.8-2.0)	
5. Colon (1.8)	
6. Lung (1.2-1.8)	
7. Esophagus (1.4)	
8. Kidney (1.5)	
9. Liver (2.7)	
10. Salivary gland (2.0)	
11. Testes (2.1)	

a. Data obtained from reference 24
b. Numbers in parentheses are the dose reduction factors or factor increases in resistance associated with WR-2721 injection.

TABLE 2

SUMMARY DATA ON THE ABILITY OF 16 EXPERIMENTAL TUMORS
TO BE PROTECTED BY OR TO ABSORB WR-2721[a]

TUMOR	PROTECTED BY WR-2721	ABSORBS SIGNIFICANT[b] QUANTITY OF WR-2721
3M2N mammary SCC[c]	No	No
R3230AC mammary AdCa	No	No
DMBA-1 mammary AdCa	No	No
13762 mammary AdCa	No	No
RFT tumor	__d	No
Morris 7777 hepatoma	—	Yes
Spont. C57 mammary Ca	No	—
C3H Fsa	No	—
KHT Sa	No	—
EMT6 mammary tumor	No	No
P-1798 LSa (solid)	—	No
CA-755 AdCa	—	No
Line 1 lung AdCa	No	No
MCa-11 mammary Ca	No	No
Urethane-induced lung Ad	No	No

a. Data obtained from reference 24
b. Significant quantities defined as greater than one-third the concentration
    of the poorest absorbing normal tissue.
c. SCC = squamous cell carcinoma; Ad = adenoma; Ca = carcinoma; FSa = fi-
    brosarcoma; Sa = sarcoma; LSa = lymphosarcoma.
d. (—) = not tested.

TABLE 3

EFFECT OF WR-2721 ON MAXIMUM TOLERABLE X-RAY DOSE & BONE MARROW RECOVERY TIME

BODY REGION	LIMITING ORGAN OR TISSUE	MAX. TOLERABLE X-RAY DOSE[a]		BONE MARROW RECOVERY TIME	
		- WR-2721	+ WR-2721	- WR-2721	+ WR-2721
Whole Body	Bone Marrow	200-300 r			
Half Body		600-700 r			
Thorax	Lung	2000 r 175 r/day	3800 r 300 r/day	6-8 wks.	2-3 wks.
Abdomen	Kidney, Colon & sm. intestine	2000 r 175 r/day	3000 r 300 r/day	6-8 wks.	2-3 wks.

a. Total (protracted) or daily

There is evidence in the literature that tri-modality therapy
combining hyperthermia, x-irradiation, and drugs which are both
radiation and heat hypoxic cell sensitizers (e.g. Nitroimidazoles
such as Metronidazole or Misonidazole; and glucose analogues such
as 5-thio-D-glucose or 2-deoxy-D-glucose) is dramatically more
effective than dual modality therapy. For example, Goldfeder et
al. (4) have demonstrated a significant therapeutic enhancement
for the mouse MT-2 mammary adenocarcinoma treated with combined
X-rays, hyperthermia (27 min. at 42.5 C during irradiation) and
misonidazole (0.67 mg/g i.p. 30 min. prior to X-rays). The number
of animals alive 4 months after treatment (11/12) as well as the
number of tumors completely regressed (9/12) was dramatically higher
in the group treated with the tri-modality regimen (see Table 4).
Hofer et al. (6) have recently shown that in vivo radiosensitization
by combined treatment with misonidazole (0.5 mg/g i.p.) and hyperthermia (45 min. at 41.5C) is dramatic in BP-8 murine sarcoma
cells (DMF=4.3) while reduced or absent in normal mouse body tissues
such as skin (DMF=1.57), intestine (DMF-1.0), or bone marrow (DMF-
1.0).

Results similar to the above have also been obtained with the
drug 5-thio-D-glucose, a glucose analogue which inhibits tumor cell
glycolysis. Song et al. (17) have shown that the cure rate of a
mouse mammary carcinoma after treatment with radiation (4500r) in
combination with hyperthermia (2 hr. at 41C) was increased from
5.8% to 53.1% when 1.5g/kg of 5-thio-D-glucose i.p. was included
in the treatment (see Fig. 1). There was no normal tissue damage
at this drug dose (L.D.-50 is 5.5.g/kg). Recent experiments (16)
have shown that 5-thio-D-glucose protects normal tissues in mice
from X-ray damage. Dose modification factors (protection) for bone
marrow and G. I. death were 1.2-1.3. while for foot skin the protection factor was 1.3 - 1.4.

One major benefit of tri-modality approaches is that therapeutic
levels of drug, X-rays, and heat can be reduced significantly and
hopefully be non-toxic. In fact, treatment at 41-42C looms especially important in view of recent observations that systemic
temperatures can rise to precarious levels (40-42C) during deep
regional heating (especially of well vascularized tumors) at 43-
45C. A question which needs to be answered is what effect WR-2721
will have on the pharmacology of a drug such as misonidazole or
5-thio-D-glucose and vice-versa. Other promising drugs which are
both heat and radiation cell sensitizers but which have yet to be
studied in tri-modality combination are the local anaesthetics
(e.g. lidocaine, procaine, xylocaine) (22) and Diethyldithiocarba-
mate, an inhibitor of Cu-superoxide dismutase (12).

Determination of an optimum fractionation and timing schedule
for sequential regional therapy combining hyperhtermia, radiation,
WR-2721 and a radio/thermo-sensitizer will depend on several factors

TABLE 4

EFFECT OF HEAT + X-RAYS + MISONIDAZOLE ON TUMOR CURE AND ANIMAL SURVIVAL[a]

TREATMENT GROUP	NO. OF ANIMALS AT START OF EX- PERIMENT	NO. OF ANIMALS ALIVE AT DAY 120	NO. OF ANIMALS WITH NONPALPABLE TUMORS	NO. OF ANIMALS WITH PALPABLE TUMORS 0.04 CU CM
Untreated con- trols[b]	12	0	0	0
X-rays alone	12	3	0	2
X-rays + 42.5°	12	4	1	0
X-rays + misoni- dazole	12	5	1	2
X-rays + 42.5° + misonidazole	12	11	9	0

a. Data obtained from reference 4
b. Mean survival time from Day 0 for the untreated controls, 23.6 ± 9.9 days.

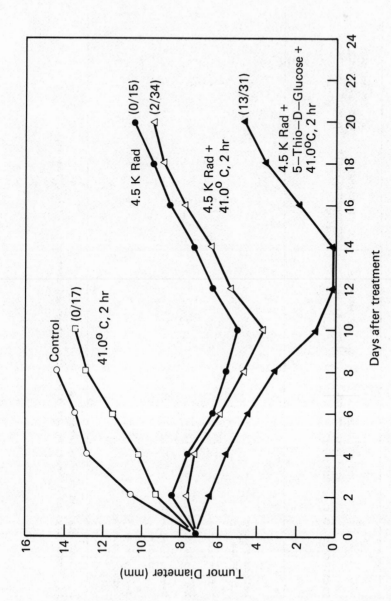

Figure 1.   Effect of heat + X-rays + 5-thio-D-glucose on tumor regression
and tumor cure (redrawn from reference 17). The fraction of
tumors cured is shown in parentheses. The tumors completely
regressed were excluded from the computation of tumor diameter
during the regrowth phase.

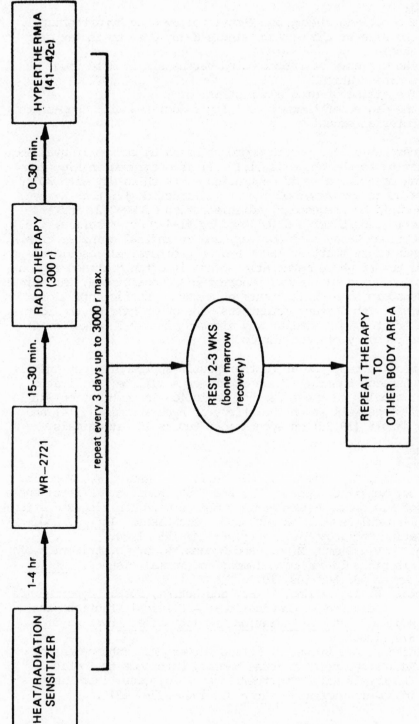

Figure 2. Therapeutic rationale for treatment of metastatic cancer incorporating sequential regional hyperthermia in combination with x-rays and heat/radiation sensitizing drug.

including:
1. The optimum timing for X-rays followed by hyperthermia.
2. The size of the maximum single X-ray dose to thorax or abdomen.
3. The efficacy of fractionated versus single dose drug administration.
4. The timing of drug administration.
4. The degree of thermal toxicity associated with deep-seated internal organs.

A reasonable therapeutic approach based on currently available data relating to the above (2,11,15,21) is diagramed in Fig. 2. The thorax or abdomen would be treated every third day with 300 r of X-rays up to a maximum of 3000 r (10 fractions). Each X-ray fraction would be preceded by administration of WR-2721 and a radio/thermo-sensitizer and followed by 41-42C hyperthermia. 300 r is an optimum X-ray dose however, and in initial clinical trials, X-ray doses might start at 150 r and be progressively escalated. For those tumors whose metastatic spread is often confined region-ally (e.g. ovarian carcinoma, pancreatic adenocarcinoma, intestinal tract adenocarcinoma) this treatment might be sufficient. For those tumors with distant metastases, the other half of the body could be treated in a similar way after a time (2-3 weeks) suffi-cient for recovery of bone-morrow.

We plan to test the above therapeutic approach in pet animals with spontaneous tumors. These experiments will be facilitated by recent studies on the effect of radiation in combination with WR-2721 (18) as well as on the effect of hyperthermia (5,14) and of Misonidazole (19,20) on spontaneous tumors in pet animals.

References

1. Arcangeli, G., Barni, E., Cividalli, A., Mauro, F., Morelli, D., Nervi, C., Spano, M., and Tabocchini, A. Effectiveness of Microwave Hyperthermia Combined with Ionizing Radiation: Clinical Results on Neck Node Metastases. Int. J. Radiation Oncology Biol. Phys. 6: 143-148, 1980.
2. Ash, D. V., Smith, M. R., and Bugden, R. D. Distribution of Misonidazole in Human Tumors and Normal Tissues. Br. J. Cancer 39: 503-509, 1979.
3. Bicher, H. I., Sandhu, T. S., and Hetzel, F. W. Hyperthermia and Radiation in Combination: A Clinical Fractionation Regime. Int. J. Radiation Oncology Biol. Phys. 6: 867-870, 1980.
4. Goldfeder, A., Brown, D. M. and Berger, A. Enhancement of Radioresponse of a Mouse Mammary Carcinoma to Combined Treatments with Hyperthermia and Radiosensitizer Mison-idazole. Cancer Research 39: 2966-2970, 1979.

5. Grier, R. L., Brewer, W. G., and Theilen, G. H. Hyperthermic Treatment of Superficial Tumors in Cats and Dogs. J. Amer. Veter. Med. Assoc. 177: 227-233, 1980.

6. Hofer, K. G., MacKinnon, A. R., Schubert, A. L., Lehr, J. E. and Grimmett, E. V. Radiosensitization of Tumors and Normal Tissues by Combined Treatment with Misonidazole and Heat. Submitted for publication, 1981.

7. Holt, J. A. G. Alternative Therapy for Recurrent Hodgkins Disease. British J. Radiology 53: 1061-1067, 1980.

8. Hornback, N. O., Shupe, R. E., Shidnia, H., Joe, B. T., Sayoc, E. and Marshall, C. Preliminary Clinical Results of Combined 433 Megahertz Microwave Therapy and Radiation Therapy on Patients with Advanced Cancer. Cancer 40: 2854-2863, 1977.

9. Kim, J. H., Hahn, E. W., and Tokita, N. Combination Hyperthermia and Radiation Therapy for Cutaneous Malignant Melanoma. Cancer 41: 2143-2148, 1978.

10. Kligerman, M. M., Shaw, M. T., Slavik, M. and Yuhas, J. M. Phase I Clinical Studies with WR-2721. Cancer Clin. Trials 3: 217-221, 1980.

11. Landau, B. R., Laszlo, J. S., Stengle, J. and Burk, D. Certain Metabolic and Pharmacologic Effects in Cancer Patients Given Infusions of 2-Deoxy-D-Glucose. J. Natl. Cancer Inst. 21: 485-494, 1958.

12. Lin, P. S., Kwock, L. and Butterfield, C. E. Diethyldithio-carbamate Enhancement of Radiation and Hyperthermic Effects on Chinese Hamster Cells in Vitro. Radiation Research 77: 501-511, 1979.

13. Marmor, J. B. and Hahn, G. M. Combined Radiation and Hyperthermia in Superficial Human Tumors. Cancer 46: 1986-1991, 1980.

14. Marmor, J. B., Pounds, D., Hahn, N. and Hahn, G. M. Treating Spontaneous Tumors in Dogs and Cats by Ultrasound-Induced Hyperthermia. Int. J. Radiation Oncology Biol. Phys. 4: 967-973, 1978.

15. Phillips, T. L. Rationale for Initial Clinical Trials and Future Development of Radioprotectors. Cancer Clin. Trials 3: 165-173, 1980.

16. Schuman, V., Song, C. W., Levitt, S. H. Radioprotective Effect of 5-Thio-D-Glucose on Normal Tissues. Abstracts of Papers For The 29th Meeting of the Radiation Research Society, 1981, p. 89.

17. Song, C. W., Kang, M. S., Stettner, S. L., and Levitt, S. H. In Vivo Effect of 5-Thio-D-Glucose on Tumor. In Radiation Sensitizers: Their Use in the Clinical Management of Cancer, L. Brady (Ed.), Masson Publishers, New York, 1980, pp. 296-301.

18. Thrall, D. E., Biery, D. N. and Girardi, A. J. Evaluation of Radiation and WR-2721 in Dogs with Spontaneous Tumors. In Radiation Sensitizers: Their Use in the Clinical Manage-

ment of Cancer, L. Brady (Ed.), Masson Publishers, New
York, 1980, pp. 343-347.

19. White, R. A. S., Workman, P., Owen, L. N. and Bleehen, N. M.
The Penetration of Misonidazole into Spontaneous Canine
Tumors. Br. J. Cancer 40: 284-293, 1979.

20. White, R. A. S., Workman, P., Freedman, L. S., Owen, L. N. and
Bleehen, N. M. The Pharmacokinetics of Misonidazole in the
Dog. Europ. J. Cancer 15: 1233-1242, 1979.

21. Wasserman, T. H., Stetz, J. and Phillips, T. L. Radiation
Therapy Oncology Group Clinical Trials with Misonidazole.
Cancer 47: 2382-2390, 1981.

22. Yau, T. M., and Kim, S. C. Local Anaesthetics as Hypoxic
Radiosensitizers, Oxic Radioprotectors and Potentiators
of Hyperthermic Killing in Mammalian Cells. British J.
Radiology 53: 587-692, 1980.

23. Yuhas, J. M. A More General Role For WR-2721 in Cancer Therapy
Br. J. Cancer 41: 832-834, 1980.

24. Yuhas, J. M., Spellman, J. M. and Culo F. The Role of WR-2721
in Radiotherapy and/or Chemotherapy. Cancer Clin. Trials
3: 211-216, 1980.

EFFECTS OF HYPERTHERMIA AND HYPERGLYCEMIA ON THE METASTASES

FORMATION AND ON SURVIVAL OF RAT BEARING W256 CARCINOSARCOMA

Sudhir A. Shah, Rakesh K. Jain and Pamela L. Finney

Cancer Research Laboratory, Department of Chemical Engineering, Carnegie-Mellon University, Pittsburgh, PA 15213

Introduction and Background

The selective destructive effect of hyperthermia (temperatures $\geqslant 42^{O}C$) on a variety of malignant tumors in animals is now well documented, and there is increasing evidence that many of the findings in animal tumor systems apply to human cancer (see Milder, 1979; Jain and Gullino, 1980). Current thrust in this field is directed towards defining the place of hyperthermia in human cancer therapy, and advance in this direction depends upon determining how best to apply and control the heat, as well as understanding more about its mechanism of action. It has been suspected for a long time that the interplay of various physiological factors (e.g. cell pH, tumor blood flow and the host immune system) other than the degree of physical heat applied may determine the outcome for a tumor treated by hyperthermia in vivo. Results to date indicate that tumors fall into two zones of thermal sensitivity, 42-43°C and 45-50°C. Most human tumors are not sensitive to 42-43°C temperature range (see Dickson and Shah, 1977), and temperatures greater than 42°C for prolonged periods can cause irreversible damage to normal surrounding tissues. Also, due to physiological limitations, disseminated disease cannot be treated by whole-body hyperthermia in the higher temperature zone. Therefore, effective treatment of cancer by hyperthermia would depend on selectively heating the tumor by manipulating tumor blood flow and by using potentiators of hyperthermia.

Stimulation of the destructive effects of hyperthermia by drugs (Overgaard, 1976; Marmor et al., 1979) radiation (Brenner and Yerushalmi, 1975; Kim et al., 1978; Hahn et al., 1979) and immunostimulants like serotonin (Crile, 1962) and Corynebacterium parvum (Urano et al., 1978, 1979; Szmigielski and Janiak, 1978; Shaw & Dickson, 1981) have been described. Von Ardenne (1970, 1972) has suggested that hyperglycemia or blood glucose levels of > 400 mg% could lead to increased tumor glycolysis, accumulation of lactic acid due to inhibition of blood flow in tumor, decrease in tumor pH and consequently increased sensitivity of cancer cells to hyperthermia. Since our previous work showed that regression of distant metastases can occur after local tumor heating (Shah and Dickson, 1978b, Shah, 1981) and that glucose loading of the host can lead to complete inhibition of tumor blood flow (Shah et al., 1981), we decided to investigate the effects of combined local hyperthermia and hyperglycemia on metastases formation and on survival of rats bearing W256 carcinosarcoma. The W256 investigated in the present work was highly malignant, spontaneous in origin (non-immunogenic) and relatively insensitive to hyperthermia (Johnson, 1940) like many human tumors.

Experimental Procedures

Tumor System. Sprague-Dawley female rats (175-200 g) were purchased from Harlan Sprague-Dawley, Madison, Wisconsin. The W256 carcinosarcoma was kindly supplied by the Mason Research Institute, Worchester, Massachusetts. W256 tumor was induced in rats by s.c. injection of 50 mg tumor slices in the dorsum of the left hind foot. Tumor volumes were calculated from caliper measurements made in the anteroposterior, lateral, and verticle planes of the foot, allowance being made for the normal foot thickness before inoculation of tumor.

Hyperglycemia. Initially, a glucose tolerance test was performed in rats by giving a single i.p. injection at 6 g/kg and 12 g/kg body weight. All rats survived this treatment. Since our previous work had shown that 6 g/kg glucose dose inhibited tumor blood flow in W256 (Shah et al., 1981), we selected this glucose dose for the present study.

Glucose and Lactate Determinations. Blood glucose was measured by glucose oxidase test kit (Boehringer Corp., Indianapolis, Indiana). Blood (0.1 ml) was taken from the jugular vein of the animal and deproteinized by adding 0.16% uranyl acetate (1 ml). Glucose was estimated by spectrophotometry at 505 nm. For tumor glucose determination, 0.3 - 0.5 g tumor tissue was homogenized in distilled water (3 ml), and the homogenate (0.5 ml) was added to 0.16% uranyl acetate (1 ml) for deproteinization. The solution was mixed well and centrifuged at 3000 r.p.m. for 10 minutes, and glucose was estimated in 0.1 ml of supernatant. Results were expressed as mg glucose in 100 ml of blood or in 100 g tumor tissue.

Blood lactate was estimated by lactate dehydrogenase oxidation

test kit (Lactate UV method; Boehringer Corp., Indianapolis,
Indiana). Blood (0.5 ml) from jugular vein was deproteinized in
0.6 N perchloric acid (1 ml). Lactate was determined by spectrophotometry at 340 nm. For tumor lactate determination, W256 was
homogenized and the homogenate (0.1 ml) was deproteinized in 0.6N
perchloric acid (1 ml). The mixture was centrifuged as above and
0.3 ml of supernatant was used for assay. Results were expressed
as mg lactate in 100 ml blood or in 100 g tumor tissue.

Hyperthermic Treatment of the W256 Tumor. Water Bath: The
heating bath consisted of an aquarium (61x31x31 cm) containing
67.5 l water heated by a thermomix 1460 circulating heater (Type
850053, number 473; VWR scientific, B. Braum Co., Pittsburgh,
Pennsylvania) with an output of 13 l/min. The unit maintained the
bath temperature constant to + 0.005°C. Initially, this aquarium
had a plexiglass (Trademark of Dupont Chemical Co. for poly-
methylmethacrylate) platform with 2 slits (3 cm wide) which could
be used for heating either foot or thigh tumors in rats. This
platform alone proved inadequate for heating foot tumors since rats
thigh often slipped into the water which elivated the body temperature and resulted in high mortality rate for animals. This platform was therefore redesigned to provide insulation for rats and
for eliminating the heating of thigh muscle. The platform was
covered with plywood containing 2.5 cm circular holes which allowed
only the foot tumors to slip into the water bath. The holes were
large enough to remove the foot out of the waterbath even after
severe edema that occured after tumor heating at 43°C for 2 hours.

Temperature Measurement: Temperatures were monitored by thermocouple probes (Omega Engineering Inc., Stamford, Connecticut)
and a 5-channel direct-reading digital light meter (Trendicator
412A, Doric Instruments, San Diego, California). For intra-tumor
temperature measurements, probes used were 1.5 cm long, needle type
HYP-1, 0.3 mm in diameter. Omega's sub-miniature thermocouple
probes (SCPSS-062G-48) were used for rectal recordings. The Doric
light meter had an accuracy of + 0.1°C. The temperature probes
were standardized against a mercury-in-glass thermometer that met
NBS specification (15-043B; Fisher Scientific Co., Pittsburgh,
Pennsylvania) and the probes were checked for "drift" before each
day's experiment.

Tumor Heating: All experiments were performed in a temperature
controlled room at 23°C. For heat treatment of foot tumors (0.8-
1.0 ml), the rats were anesthetized with 0.1 ml of 1:4 dilution of
Nembutal veterinary given i.p. (50 mg pentobarbitone sodium per ml;
Abbott Laboratories, North Chicago, Illinois 60064) per 50 g body
weight. Narcosis was maintained by further i.p. injections of 0.1
ml of Nembutal as needed. For intratumor temperature measurements,
thermocouple needle was inserted in the center of the tumor mass
(see Fig. 1). Up to 10 tumor-bearing rats were set up on the plexi-

glass platform (see Fig. 2) and intratumor temperature was elevated
to 43°C for 2 hours. Tumor temperature was maintained to within
+ 0.1°C and readings taken at 8-10 minute intervals on the Doric
light meter. The instrument had a fast response time of 2 seconds
and was unaffected by changes in ambient temperature. Immediately
after heat treatment, each rat was given 1 ml of normal saline
(0.9% NaCl) to replace fluid loss. The rats were wraped in a
blanket and placed under a table lamp to prevent an overswing of
body temperature to subnormal levels; this can occur rapidly in
rats following hyperthermia.

Results

    The administration of glucose (6g/kg body weight, i.p.) caused
a rise in the blood glucose levels from 135 mg% (+ 10 mg%, S.D.)
to 690 mg% (+ 50 mg%, S.D.) within 1 hour after injection (Fig. 3).
A mean of about 500 mg% was maintained during the heat treatment
period, between 2-4 hours. The blood glucose level fell steadily
from 1 hour to 5 hours (250 mg% + 55 mg%) and then remained at this
level for at least a further 1½ hour. The normal tumor glucose
level was about 15 mg% (+ 5 mg%, S.D.). This increased to 300 mg%
(+ 30 mg%, S.D.) within 1 hour after glucose loading and remained
at between 110 - 150 mg% level for up to 6½ hours.

    Figure 4 details the effect of glucose loading on blood and
tumor lactate levels. Blood lactate levels remained unaltered, at
25 mg% (+ 20 mg%, S.D.), after glucose injection to rats. The
tumor lactate levels increased five fold to 125 mg% (+ 50 mg%, S.D.)
by 3 hours after glucose administration. This level then declined
slowly to 60 mg% (+ 40 mg%, S.D.) by 6½ hours. The mean tumor
lactate level during the heat treatment (2-4 hours) was approximately
87 mg%, i.e. about double the normal level.

    Text figure 5 shows the temperature gradient between normo-
glycemic and hyperglycemic W256 tumors and the water-bath during
heat treatment at 43°C. The hyperglycemic tumors showed a smaller
temperature gradient throughout the heating period. The mean
difference in the temperature gradient between normal and hyperglycemic tumors was about 1°C for the first 70 minutes in the water
bath. This difference decreased steadily thereafter and was 0.1°C
by 2 hours after starting the heat treatment.

    Figure 6 illustrates the effect of local heating on primary
tumor volumes in untreated and heat treated rats. From an initial
transplant of 50 mg tumor into the left hind foot of the rat, the
tumor reached a volume of 0.8-1.0 ml by 5 days. Untreated, the
tumors increased in volume exponentially to 4.56 ml (+ 1 ml, S.D.)
by 12 days after implantation. Seventy seven percent of the untreated rats died by 15 days. Hyperglycemia lead to restraint in
tumor growth and 27% of rats showed spontaneous regression by 30

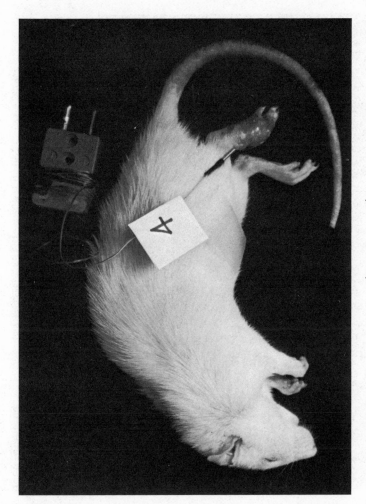

Figure 1 Rat showing W256 foot tumor (0.8-1.0 ml) on day 5 after s.c. injection of 50 mg tumor slices. Intratumor temperature during heat treatment was measured with needle thermocouple connected to digital Doric light meter.

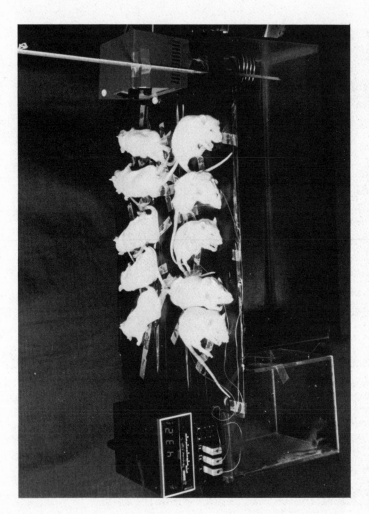

Figure 2 Experimental arrangement for heating rat foot tumors (0.8-1.0 ml) by water
bath immersion at 43OC for 2 hours. Animals are anesthetized with Nembutal
veterinary given i.p. and placed on plexiglass platform resting over the water
bath. Tumor bearing foot is immersed in the water through a 2.5 cm diameter
padded opening. Intratumor temperature during heat treatment is continuously
monitored by needle thermocouple probes connected to a 5-channel digital Doric
light meter.

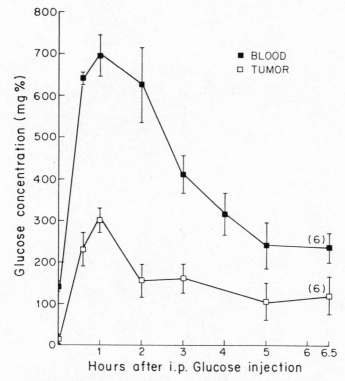

Figure 3 Blood and tumor (0.8-1.0 ml) glucose concentrations in anesthetized tumor-bearing rats after i.p. glucose (6g-kg) injection. Glucose was measured by the glucose oxidase test kit. Each point for blood or tumor glucose was the mean +S.D. from 3-5 rats. Data for time 0 were obtained from 6-8 untreated animals.

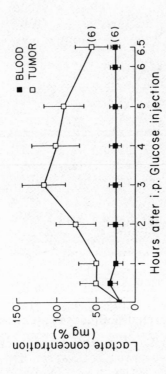

Figure 4 Blood and tumor (0.8–1.0 ml) lactate concentrations in anesthetized tumor-bearing rats after i.p. glucose (6g/kg) injection. Lactate was measured by the lactate dehydrogenase oxidation method. Each point is the mean + S.D. from 3–5 rats. Mean lactate at time 0 was obtained from 6–8 untreated animals.

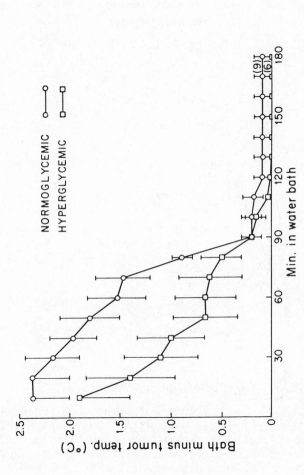

Figure 5 Simultaneously recorded bath and intratumor temperatures by needle thermocouples in normoglycemic and hyperglycemic (6g glucose/kg, i.p.) foot-tumor bearing rats during tumor heating at 43°C. The animals were treated by water bath hyperthermia 1 hour after glucose injection. The numbers in parentheses denotes the number of tumor (animals) studied in each group of rats.

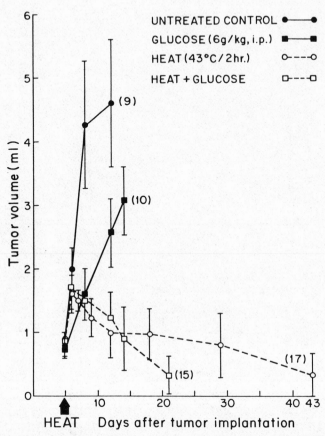

Figure 6 Changes in W256 tumor volume following combined hyperthermia
and hyperglycemia. Five days after tumor implant, the
tumor (0.8-1.0 ml) was treated by water bath immersion at
43°C for 2 hours. Tumor volumes for the growth curve were
obtained from caliper measurements. For combined treatment, glucose (6g/kg) was given to rats 1 hour before
thermotherapy. The numbers in parentheses denotes the
number of tumors (animals) treated in each group.

days. The other 73% of animals died by 15 days. Local heating at
43°C for 2 hours lead to a rapid decline in tumor volume in all 17
rats. The primary tumors regressed faster in rats treated by
hyperglycemia, but most rats died with wide spread metastases as
discussed below.

Figure 7 summarizes the tumor/host cure rates in untreated and
in heat treated animals. Of the 17 rats treated by hyperthermia
alone, 5 (30%) showed complete tumor regression by 21 days post-
heating. Seven of 17 rats (41%) were alive 38 days after hyperthermia. The animal survival after thermotherapy therefore increased
from 23% to 41% when compared to untreated control rats. Combined
hyperthermia and hyperglycemia decreased the tumor cure rate to
16% (4 of 25) and the animal survival rate to 12% (3 of 25).

Figure 8 compares the frequency of tissue involvement by W256
tumor metastases in different groups of rats. Following implantation
of tumor into the foot, 75% of the control untreated rats that died
by 15 days showed macroscopic metastases (tumor nodules) in iliac
and inguinal lymph nodes and in lungs. No tumor involvement of
either kidneys or of eyes was found. Metastases were less frequent
in animals that died following primary tumor heating. Lymph nodes
and lungs were involved with tumor in 36% of the heat treated rats.
Nine percent of these rats also showed the presense of tumor nodues
in the right kidney. In hyperglycemic rats, the frequency of tumor
involvement of lymph nodes, lungs and kidneys was greater than in
either untreated control rats or after hyperthermia alone. At post-
mortem, 80-86% rats had tumor in iliac and inguinal lymph nodes
and lungs, and 33% animals showed a large tumor mass in the posterior
abdominal wall surrounding the right kidney (Fig. 9).

Discussion

The results demonstrated that local heating of W256 carcinosarcoma by waterbath immersion at 43°C for 2 hours increased the
survival rate of animals from 23% to 41% with concomitant decrease
in the metastases formation in lungs and lymph nodes. Hyperglycemia
or blood glucose level of about 500 mg% rendered foot tumors
physically more easy to heat. However, the combined treatment
decreased the survival rate of animals to 12%, and most rats died
with increased spread of metastases in lymph nodes, lungs and
especially in the abdominal cavity involving the right kidney.

It was first postulated by Von Ardenne (1970, 1972) that hyperglycemia or blood glucose level of between 300-500 mg% may
potentiate the destructive effects of hyperthermia on tumors. He
claimed that hyperglycemia would lead to increased tumor glycolysis,
accumulation of lactic acid due to inhibition of tumor blood flow,
and consequently "optimized tumor hyperacidity" resulting in decreased tumor pH. The decreased tumor pH would cause labiliza-

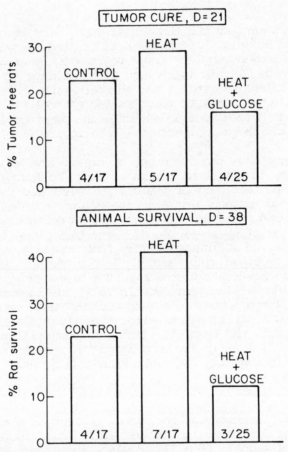

Figure 7 Effect of combined hyperthermia and hyperglycemia on W256
tumor cure and animal survival. The foot tumors (0.8-1.0
ml) were treated by water bath heating at 43°C for 2 hours
on fifth day after implantation. Hyperglycemia was induced
as described in Fig. 6. Figures within histograms indicate
number of tumor free (top histograms, day 21 post-heating)
or number of surviving animals (bottom histograms, day 38
post-heating) over total number of rats in each group under
study.

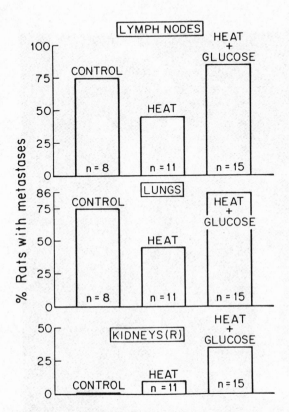

Figure 8 Frequency of tissue involvement by metastases following
combined hyperthermia and hyperglycemia in rats. Tumor
bearing animals were treated as described in Figs. 6 and
7. The percentage of rats with metastases in different
organs were calculated from numbers of animals showing
gross macroscopic tumor involvement over total number of
post-mortems performed for each group of animals (i.e.
numbers shown within the histograms).

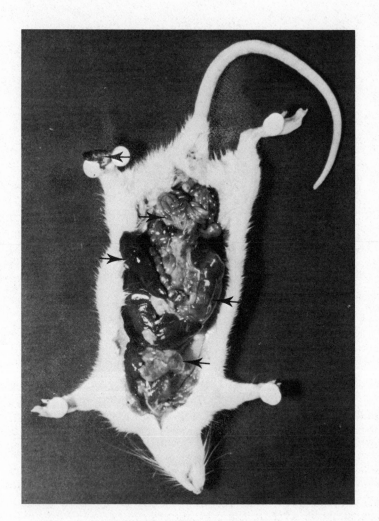

Figure 9   Gross enlargement of the spleen and kidney by W256 tumor. The primary tumor (0.8-1.0 ml) in the left foot was heated at 43°C for 2 hours on day 5 after tumor implant in hyperglycemic rat. The animal died 28 days later. At autopsy, the abdomen was full of serosanguineous fluid, a large mass of tumor occupied the abdominal cavity, surrounded and involved the right kidney, and bound the coils of the small intestine together; lung was also partially replaced by tumor.

tion of the lysozomal membrane and release of hydrolytic enzymes
which would destroy cancer cells. Von Ardenne (1970, 1972) suggested
that the tumor autolysis would begin at pH 6.7-6.8 with optimal
effects at between pH 6-6.5: and elevated temperature as low as
40°C would be effective in tumor destruction. In the present work,
glucose loading (blood glucose levels of 520 mg%) of W256 tumor
bearing rats lead to a 3-4 fold increase in tumor lactic acid
concentration (Fig. 4). Our previous work showed that hyperglycemia inhibits blood flow in W256 (Jain et al, 1979: Shah et al
1981) and there are indications that it also decreased the tumor
pH from about 7.2 to 6.6, as measured in the tumor interstitial
fluid in vivo (Shah and Jain, unpublished work). Depsite these
favorable changes in the tumor, hyperglycemia failed to potentiate
the effects of hyperthermia, therefore, our results do not support
the postulate of Von Ardenne (1970, 1972). It should be noted
that Schloerb et al (1965) failed to produce intracellular acidosis
by administering glucose (6g/kg body weight) in W256 bearing rats.
Three hours after glucose loading, a slight rise in intracellular
pH, as measured by a chemical method, from 7.19 to 7.36 was observed.
With W256 tumor slices in vitro Hult and Larson (1976) also observed
an increase in the intracellular pH from 7.12 to up to 7.51 within
5 minutes of addition of glucose (25 mM). It may be argued that
potentiation of heat therapy by hyperglycemia did not occur in the
present work because intracellular pH of W256 tumor may not have
been affected. In this respect, hyperglycemia has been shown to
potentiate the effects of hyperthermia (42° C/3 hours) for a rat
Mc7 sarcoma in which a decrease in both extracellular and intracellular pH was observed; but not in rats bearing Yoshida sarcoma
in which extracellular pH fell from 7.2 to 6.6 and intracellular
pH increased from 7.2 to 7.4 (Jackson and Dickson, 1979).

    Dickson and Calderwood (1979, 1980) have recently examined
Von Ardenne's postulate in depth using rat Yoshida sarcoma as a
tumor model. Hyperglycemia (6g glucose/kg body weight, blood
glucose level of 400-500 mg%) lead to a decrease in extracellular
pH, as measured by miniature glass capillary electrodes, from 7.2
to 6.6 within 4 hours. The intracellular pH, however, was not
significantly affected. Respiration and glycolysis of Yoshida
tumor slices from hyperglycemic rats was completely inhibited at
40°C in vitro, and the effect was equivalent to heat alone at 42°C.
However, tumor heating at 40°C in hyperglycemic host was not
equivalent to hyperthermia at 42°C (Dickson and Calderwood, 1979).
Yoshida sarcoma (1-1.5 ml foot tumors) could be cured in 100% of
the rats following local hyperthermia at 42°C for 1 hour. When
heat was applied 4 hours after hyperglycemia, there was no apparent
effect on tumor regression and animal cure was unaltered. With a
small number of rats, tumor heating at 42°C for 45 minutes itself
gave no tumor regression, 80% of tumors regressed with host cure
when hyperglycemic animals underwent heat treatment, however.
Continuous glucose infusion (blood glucose levels of 1000 mg%) for

4 hours followed by hyperthermia at 42°C for 1 hour lead to death
in 66% of the treated rats; most rats died with widespread metastases. These results were attributed by the authors to the difference in the host response to 500 mg% versus 1000 mg% blood glucose
levels. Dickson and Calderwood (1980) suggested that total inhibition of tumor blood flow is undesirable since effective immune
response to tumor would require access of lymphocytes and/or macrophages and egress of such cells and also possibly egress of breakdown products from the heated tumor.

     Several studies have recently shown that host immunocompetence
can be stimulated by effective local tumor heating. Thus, in
rabbit VX2 carcinoma (Shah, 1977; Shah and Dickson, 1978a,b) rat
Mc7 sarcoma (Shah and Dickson, 1981) and rat Guerin carcinoma
(Szmigielski and Janiak, 1978) tumor systems, tumor-regression after
local heating was accompanied by increased cellular and humoral
immunocompetence. Animals that failed to respond to heat treatment
showed decreased immunocompetence as the tumor increased in volume
with time. The immune tests employed for detecting anti-tumor
activity of the host animal were delayed hypersensitivity skin tests
against tumor extracts, estimations of anti-tumor anti-body in serum
and lymphocyte cytotoxicity against tumor cells in vitro. The
augmented response of the animal to foreign antigens was monitored
by skin testing with DNCB, lymphocyte stimulation with phyto-
hemagglutinin and antibody response to bovine serum albumin. When
the immunocompetence of animals was depressed by whole-body irradiation plus cortisone acetate, tumor failed to regress after curative
heat therapy and the host cure rate decreased. An intact host
immune response therefore appears to be necessary in order to obtain
maximum benefit from tumor heating. Some animal data further
suggests that host response to hyperthermia may be non-specific in
nature mainly involving macrophages of the reticuloendothelial
system. Impairment of host macrophage function by silica or non-
specific stimulation of its activity by Corynebacterium parvum has
been shown to significantly affect tumor response to hyperthermia
(Szmigielski and Janiak, 1978; Urano et al, 1978; Shah and Dickson,
1979; Urano et al, 1979; Shah, 1981; Shah and Dickson, 1981;
Alfieri et al, 1981). To date, Corynebacterium parvum, a non-
specific immuno stimulant, has proved to be a powerful potentiator
of hyperthermia and this agent should be further investigated with
a variety of transplantable and specially spontaneous animal tumors
which are non-immunogenic like human cancers.

     Evidence in favor of immune response after local tumor heating
in patients is mostly circumstantial except one report (Stehlin
et al, 1975) where increased lymphocyte and plasma cytotoxicity
against autologous tumor cells have been reported for patients with
melanoma treated by hyperthermic perfusion at 40°C with L-phenyla-
lanine mustard (melphalan). These various findings, mainly in
animal tumor systems, therefore, strongly suggests that host immune

system play a central role in tumor regression by hyperthermia. Agents like glucose which inhibits tumor blood flow may interfere with an effective host immune response against primary tumor and against distant metastases.

In conclusion, many animal and human tumors, like the W256 carcinosarcoma studied here, are insensitive to hyperthermia in 42-43°C temperature range (see Dickson and Shah, 1977). For W256, Johnson (1940) reported a 50% host cure after tumor heating at 43.5°C for as much as 6 hours with short radio waves. A 70% cure was achieved by heating this tumor at 47°C for 45 minutes. Radio frequency, microwave and ultrasound heating methods have been employed for treating tumors at high temperatures (see Hahn et al, 1980). However, due to irreversible damage to normal tissues, it is often not feasible to heat tumors over 43°C for prolong periods and hence potentiators are urgently needed which can be used with sub-optimal tumor heating. Rapid spread of metastases in hyperglycemic rats in the present work may have been due to "bursting out" of cancer cells from the disrupted tumor architecture by hyperthermia as blood flow returned to normal by 12 hrs. The therapeutic combination of heat and a more defined immunostimulant, such as Corynebacterium parvum (which does not affect tumor blood flow), may thus seem a local step.

Acknowledgements

This was supported by grants from NCI (CA-00643), ACS (PDT-150) and NSF (ENG-78-25432).

Summary

Hyperthermia (temperatures > 42°C) is widely used in the treatment of cancer. Current thrust in this field is directed towards using agents which can potentiate the effects of hyperthermia. Combined local hyperthermia (43°C/2 hours) and hyperglycemia (6g glucose/kg body weight; mean blood glucose levels of 500 mg%) was investigated for treating a metastasizing form of a rat W256 carcinosarcoma. Glucose loading of the tumor-bearing rats rendered the foot tumors physically more easy to heat (due to inhibition of tumor blood flow), but combined hyperthermia and hyperglycemia lead to a decrease in survival rate (13% compared to 41% with heat alone), most animals died with widespread metastases in lymph nodes, lungs and kidneys. The data does not support the postulate that hyperglycemia leads to sensitization of tumor destruction by hyperthermia. We suggest that Corynebacterium parvum, a non-specific immunostimulant, should be thoroughly investigated as a potentiator of hyperthermia.

REFERENCES

Alfieri, A. A., Hahn, E. W. and Kim, J. H. "Role of cell-
    mediated immunity in tumor eradication by hyperthermia",
    Cancer Res. 41, 1301-1305, 1981.
Brenner, H. J. and Yerushalmi, A. "Combined local hyperthermia
    and X-irradiation in the treatment of metastatic tumors",
    Br. J. Cancer 33, 91-95, 1975.
Crile, G. "Selective destruction of Cancers after exposure to
    heat", Annals of Surgery, 156, 404-407, 1962.
Dickson, J. A. and Calderwood, S. K. "Effects of hyperglycemia
    and hyperthermia on the pH, glycolysis, and respiration
    of the Yoshida sarcoma in vivo", J. Nat. Cancer Inst.,
    63, 1371-1381, 1979.
Dickson, J. A. and Calderwood, S. K. "Temperature range and
    selective sensitivity of tumors to hyperthermia: A
    Critical Review", In: R. K. Jain and P. M. Gullino (Eds.),
    "Thermal Characteristics of Tumors: Applications in
    Detection and Treatment", Ann. N.Y. Acad. Sci., 335, 180-
    205, 1980.
Dickson, J. A. and Shah, S. A. "Technology for the Hyperthermic
    Treatment of Large Solid Tumors at 50°", Clin. Oncol.
    3, 301-318, 1977.
Hahn, G. M., Kernahan, P., Martinez, A., Pounds, D. and Prionas,
    S. "Some heat transfer problems associated with heating
    by ultrasound, microwaves, or radiofrequency", In: R. K.
    Jain and P. M. Gullino (Eds.), "Thermal Characteristics
    of Tumors: Applications in Detection and Treatment",
    Ann. N.Y. Acad. Sci., 335, 327-346, 1980.
Hult, R. L. and Larson, R. E. "Dissociation of 5-Fluorouracil
    uptake from intracellular pH in Walker 256 carcinosarcoma",
    Cancer Treat. Rep., 60, 867-873, 1976.
Jackson, D. J. and Dickson, J. A. "Combination hyperthermia
    (42°C) and hyperglycemia in the treatment of the Mc7
    sarcoma", Br. J. Cancer, 40, 306, 1979.
Jain, R. K., Grantham, F. H. and Gullino, P. M. "Blood flow
    and heat transfer in Walker 256 mammary carcinoma", J.
    Natl. Cancer Inst., 62, 927-933, 1979.
Jain, R. K. and Gullino, P. M. (Eds.), "Thermal Characteristics
    of Tumors: Applications in Detection and Treatment",
    Ann. N.Y. Acad. Sci., 335, 1980.
Johnson, H. J. "The action of short radio waves on tissues.
    III. A comparison of the thermal sensitivities of
    transplantable tumors in vivo and in vitro", Am. J.
    Cancer, 38, 533-550, 1940.
Kim, J. H., Hahn, E. W. and Tokita, N. "Combination hyper-
    thermia and radiation therapy for cutaneous malignant
    melanoma", Cancer, 41, 2143-2148, 1978.
Marmor, J. B., Kozak, D. and Hahn, G. M. "Effects of systemi-
    cally administered Bleomycin or Adriamycin with local

hyperthermia on primary tumor and lung metastases",
Cancer Treat. Rep., 63, 1279-1290, 1979.

Milder, J. W. (Ed.), Conference on Hyperthermia in Cancer
Treatment Cancer Res., 39, 2232-2340, 1979.

Overgaard, J. "Combined Adriamycin and hyperthermia treatment
of a murine mammary carcinoma in vivo", Cancer Res., 36,
3077-3081, 1976.

Schloerb, P. R., Blackburn, G. L., Grantham, J. J., Mallard,
D. S. and Cage, G. K. "Intracellular pH and buffering
capacity of the Walker 256 carcinoma", Surgery, 58, 5-11,
1965.

Shah, S. A. "The influence of the Immune System on the
Response of the Rabbit VX2 Carcinoma to Hyperthermia",
Ph.D. Thesis (295 pages), Faculty of Medicine, University
of Newcastle upon Tyne, England, 1977.

Shah, S. A. "Participation of the immune system in regression
of a rat Mc7 sarcoma by hyperthermia", Cancer Res., 41,
1742-1747, 1981.

Shah, S. A. and Dickson, J. A. "Effect of hyperthermia on
the immune response of normal rabbits", Cancer Res. 38,
3518-3522, 1978a.

Shah, S. A. and Dickson, J. A. "Effect of hyperthermia on
the immunocompetence of VX2 tumor-bearing rabbits",
Cancer Res., 38, 3523-3531, 1978b.

Shah, S. A. and Dickson, J. A. "Effect of hyperthermia on the
phagocytic activity of tumor-bearing animals", Br. J.
Cancer, 40, 818-819, 1979.

Shah, S. A. and Dickson, J. A. "Influence of the macrophage
activity on the response of a rat Mc7 sarcoma to hyperthermia (43°C)", Br. J. Cancer, in press, 1981.

Shah, S. A., Finney, P. L., Malley, J. A., Hecht, D. J. and
Jain, R. K. "Modification of blood flow in W256
carcinosarcoma by hyperglycemia (HG) and hypervolemia
(HV): A thermal probe method (TPM)", In: Proc. of 72nd
Ann. Meeting of Am. Ass. Cancer Res., 22, 60, 1981.

Stehlin, F. S., Giovanella, B. C., Delpolyi, P. D., Muenz,
L. R. and Anderson R. F. "Results of hyperthermic
perfusion for melanoma of the extremities", Surg. Gynecol.
Obstet., 140, 339-348, 1975.

Szmigielski, S. and Janiak, M. "Reaction of cell-mediated
immunity to local hyperthermia of tumors and its potenti-
ation by immunostimulation", In: C. Streffer, D. Van
Beuningen, F. Dietzel, Rottinger, E., Robinson, J. E.,
Scherer, E., Seeber, S. and Trott, K. R. (Eds.),
International Symposium on Cancer Therapy by Hyperthermia
and Radiation, Essen., 1977, pp. 80-88, Baltimore: Urban
& Schwarzenberg, 1978.

Urano, M., Overgaard, M., Suit, H. D., Dunn, P. and Sedlacek,
R. S. "Enhancement by Corynebacterium parvum of the
normal and tumor tissue response to hyperthermia",

Cancer Res., 38, 862–864, 1978.

Urano, M., Suit, H. D., Dunn, P., Lansdale, T. and Sedlacek, R. S., "Enhancement of the thermal response of animal tumors by Corynebacterium parvum", Cancer Res., 39, 3454–3457, 1979.

Von Ardenne, M., Krebs-Mehrschritt-Therapie, 2 Auflage, Berlin: VEB Verlag Volk und Gesundheit, 1970.

Von Ardenne, M., "Selective multiphase cancer therapy. Conceptual aspects and experimental basis", Adv. Pharmacol. Chemother., 10, 339–380, 1972.

COMPUTER CONTROLLED HYPERTHERMIA UNIT FOR CANCER THERAPY

Juan V. Fayos, M.D., Charles F. Gottlieb, Ph.D., Young
H. Kim, M.D., and Quirino Balzano, Ph.D.*

Division of Radiation Therapy (D31), Dept. of Radiology,
University of Miami School of Medicine, P.O. Box 016960,
Miami, Florida 33101, *Motorola, Inc., 8000 W. Sunrise
Blvd., Plantation, Florida 33322

Abstract

A versatile hyperthermia control system, based on a microcomputer, provides automated temperature regluation (1 channel) and
monitoring (3 channels) and control of microwave output (both on/
off and power level), and displays temperature (^{o}C) and microwave
output (watts) graphically in real time; all data are stored on
floppy diskette.

Introduction

Hyperthermia for cancer treatment is generating considerable
interest, both as the sole form of treament and also in combination
with radiation therapy or chemotherapy (1-7). Hyperthermia has
come to mean the artificial elevation of tissue temperature above
$41^{o}C$, with therapeutic intent (1). Although hyperthermia can be
induced either locally, or to the whole body, this paper considers
only the localized version.

Factors limiting the development and reproducibility of this
form of experimental therapy include the lack of precise control
of heating, and the lack of detailed recording of such events as
the amount of heat used and the temperature, both as a function
of time. We have overcome these shortcomings. In fact, our
computerized system not only controls the heating to that required
to maintain the desired tissue temperature, but also automates
hyperthermia treatment.

Components of the system

The hyperthermia system consists of three major components, each with its related accessories, (presented in block diagram in Figure 1):
1. a dedicated microcomputer with its associated hardware and software,
2. a microwave power generator, power sensors, and applicator antenna, and
3. a thermocouple thermometry system.

Computer

The "brain" of the system is an Apple II plus microcomputer which controls the entire hyperthermia system. The computer comes with an ASCII keyboard, 8 peripheral connectors, and an input/output (I/0) connector. The I/0 connector provides analog input (resistive), and digital (single bit) I/0. Through the 8 peripheral connectors, numerous devices can be connected; those of particular significance

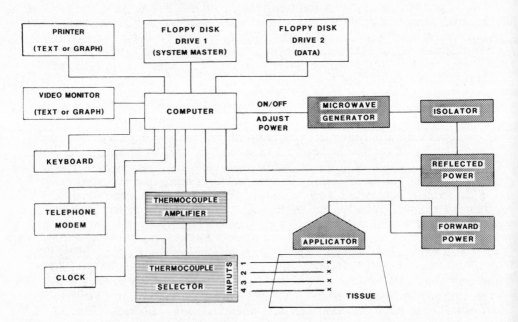

Figure 1. Block diagram of the Computer Controlled Hyperthermia System.   Microcomputer and associated hardware.   Microwave power generator, power sensors, and applicator.   Thermocouple thermometry system.

include floppy disk drives, relays, real time clock, printer, telephone modem, and additional analog (voltage) inputs. Information output from the computer (text or graph) may be displayed on a video monitor, printed, and/or stored on floopy disks.

Microwave Generator, Power Sensors, Applicator

The microwave power generator is an MCL Model 15222 RF Power Generator used with a Model 6050M plug in RF Oscillator Module, producing about 150 watts at 915 MHz, and tunable from 400 to 1000 MHz. Output is continuously adjustable from a few milliwatts to the maximum. The generator is fully software controlled, i.e., RF output is turned on and off, and the output level (when on) is adjusted.

Forward and reflected power are sensed using a pair of RF Line Section Assemblies and plug in elements, adapted from Bird THRULINE RF Directional Wattmeters (Model 43). They are calibrated so that the computer may sense forward and reflected power.

The applicator for this system consists of an air filled excitation chamber (cavity) which can operate at 150 MHz and higher frequencies, and waveguide attachments. A series of waveguides of different cross section and dielectric loading can be excited by this chamber, so as to select the most suitable applicator aperature for each tumor size, shape, and depth.

Thermocouple Thermometry

The thermometry uses a Bailey Instruments Model BAT-8C Digital Thermometer with standard Type T (copper constantan) thermocouples, and temperature compensated amplifier (external temperature reference unnecessary). The analog temperature (voltage) from the thermometer is input to the computer, which is calibrated to determine sensor temperature. Computerized switches select which of four sensors connected to the unit is measured. We are using Bailey IT-21 probes, each consisting of a minature thermocouple junction with 44 gauge (0.05 mm) leads encapsulated in teflon; the probe is inserted into tissue through a 21 gauge hypodermic needle. Any electrically isolated Type T thermocouple may be used with the system.

Electronic interference in temperature measurement is eliminated by switching the RF off for one second before reading the temperature; direct RF heating of these minature thermocouples is minimal. Comparison temperature measurements in simulated tissue were made in a high power RF field, using these thermocouples and a non-perturbing probe (Vitek Electrothermia Monitor), both with calibrations traceable to the U.S. National Bureau of Standards. The average temperature difference was 0.02°C (standard deviation 0.15°C). The maximum difference in the 25 pairs of measurements was 0.4°C.

System Operation

    System operation is highly automated. The operator inserts the
System Master and Data Diskettes into disk drives 1 and 2, respectively, and starts the computer. A "menu" is displayed, from which
the user may select from several functions (eg. hyperthermia
treatment, or a data processing option). For treatment, the software provides "default" values and queries the user for changes in
the parameters, which include: temperature to be achieved and
maintained (Channel 1), time that temperature is to be maintained,
time to monitor temperatures before and after heating, time to
raise the temperature to that prescribed, temperature limits imposed
(Channels 2-4), etc. The patient is positioned on a couch, the
thermocouples inserted as appropriate, and the applicator positioned.
The computer then executes the prescribed treatment automatically,
without operator interaction. As programed, the computer monitors
temperature, adjusts output power, turns output on and off, and
stores critical parameters of that treatment along with starting
time, temperatures and their measurement times, incident RF power
and its on and off times, etc. on the Data Diskette. The computer
also displays the temperature of each channel and the incident
microwave power (histogram, 0 to 100 watts) on the video monitor,
in real time, with updating as the treatment progresses (Figure 2).

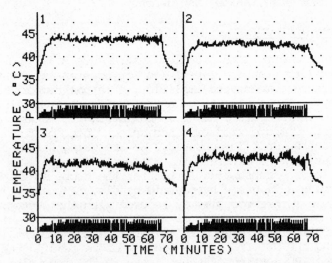

    Figure 2. Graphic data output; identical to video display
during treatment. "P" denotes incident microwave power (histogram).
Results are from hyperthermia treatment of a patient with recurrent
cervical carcinoma. The lesion was a superficial metastasis. Probe
positions: Channel 1, 1.6 cm deep in tissue; Channels 2 to 4, skin
surface within the heating field.

TABLE I

LENGTHS OF THE PHASES OF HYPERTHERMIA TREATMENT[*]

Phase of Treatment	Time (minutes)
BASELINE	0.89
RISE	7.23
TREATMENT	59.78
DECAY	8.97

[*] Same data as Figure 2. Computer programmed for 44 $^{\circ}$C (Channel 1) for 60 minutes.

TABLE II

TEMPERATURE STATISTICS ($^{\circ}$C)[*]

	Channel Number			
	1	2	3	4
Mean	43.8	42.5	41.3	42.7
Standard Deviation	0.5	0.5	0.7	0.7
Minimum	42.6	40.9	39.6	39.9
Maximum	44.9	43.6	43.3	44.4

[*] Same data as Figure 2. Computer programmed for 44 $^{\circ}$C (Channel 1) for 60 minutes.

TABLE III

MICROWAVE POWER STATISTICS[*]

	Power (watts)
Mean	71.0
Standard Deviation	15.2
Minimum	37.0
Maximum	90.0
Duty Factor	0.73

[*] Same data as Figure 2. Computer programmed for 44 $^{\circ}$C (Channel 1) for 60 minutes.

The treatment record on the Data Diskette is an inexpensive means of record storage. More than 20 treatments can be stored on a single diskette. The entire treatment can be reconstructed from the stored information, either as a tabular listing, or graph. The data may be processed to give the length of time for each of the four phases of a hyperthermia treatment (Table I), and to give the average temperature during treatment, its standard deviation and maximum and minimum values, decay of hyperthermia (thermal "wash-out"), etc., for each temperature channel (Table II). Likewise, the average incident RF power and its minimum and maximum are readily obtained (Table III). Additionally, the data may be forwarded (via the telephone modem) to large remote computers, permitting sophisticated analysis.

Advantages of this system

The advantages of this system over those previously available for hyperthermia research are numerous. Precise control of heating (tissue temperature) minimizes temperature fluctuations. The time to raise the temperature to that for hyperthermia is controlled. The floppy diskette is an inexpensive means of record storage, and the treatment may be completely reconstructed at a later time.

Aside from the more scientific attributes offered by this hyperthermia system, the complete unit was constructed for a very modest cost (less than $15,000), especially considering its sophisticated capabilities.

References

1. Short JG, Turner PF. PROC IEEE 68: 133, 1980.
2. Field SB, Bleehen NM. Cancer Treat Rev. 6: 63,1979.
3. Proc Int Symp Cancer Therapy by Hyperthermia and Radiation, Washington, D. C. Apr. 28-30, 1975. American College of Radiology, 1975.
4. Proc Second Int Symp Cancer Therapy by Hyperthermia and Radiation, Essen, Jun. 2-4, 1977. Ed. Streffer C., et al, Urban and Schwarzenberg, Baltimore, 1978.
5. Proc Third Int Symp Cancer Therapy by Hyperthermia, Drugs, and Radiation, Fort Collins, Co., Jun. 22-26, 1980. J. Natl. Cancer Inst. in press.
6. Proc First Meet Europ Group Hyperthermia in Radiation Oncology, Cambridge, Sept. 9-10, 1979. Ed. Arcangeli G, Mauro F. Masson, Milan, 1980.
7. Hand JW, ter Haar G. Brit J., Radiol 54: 443, 1981.

IMPACT OF LOCALIZED MICROWAVE HYPERTHERMIA ON THE OXYGENATION

STATUS OF MALIGNANT TUMORS*

J. Otte, R. Manz, G. Thews, and P. Vaupel

Department of Physiology, University of Mainz, D-6500
Mainz, West Germany - Department of Physiology, University
of Regensburg, D-8400 Regensburg, West Germany

Introduction

Considerable insight into the mechanisms of heat induced cell
death in vitro has been gained during recent years (for reviews
see 1-3). Besides the direct cell killing effect of heat, many
microenvironmental or milieu factors seem to play an important
role during heat treatment of solid tumors in vivo, such that a
preferential effect of hyperthermia on tumors has been postulated
for the in situ conditions. Environmental factors affecting the
tumor milieu, such as tissue oxygen partial pressures, pH values,
glucose (?) and lactate levels, nutrient supply and drainage of
wastes, have thus become a subject of topical interest.

The importance of the alterations in the microenvironment of
the tumor cells is supported by the observations that (i) chronically
hypoxic cells are more sensitive to heat than are oxygenated cells
(4,5), and (ii) low pH values increase the thermal sensitivity of
tumor cells (5,6).

The micrometabolic milieu which appears to be a critical
determinant of the response of tumors to hyperthermia is largely
determined by the efficiency of nutritive blood flow through tumors.
Some recent experimental evidence suggests that hyperthermia has
profound effects on tumor blood flow, including tumor microcirculation (7-9). Histopathological studies of hyperthermic effects
on the tumor microvasculature reveal patterns of gradual changes
which likely cause these variations in tumor blood flow (10,11).
However, pronounced heterogeneities, both temporal and spatial, in

*Supported by Deutsche Forschungsgemeinschaft (Va 57/2-1)

nutritive blood flow and in tumor temperature render general state-
ments on heat induced milieu changes more complicated.

In pursuing our own investigations of tumor blood flow and of
oxygen supply to tumors during hyperthermia, the present experiments
were undertaken in order to study the oxygenation changes in tumors.
For characterization of the oxygenation status of the tumor, the
oxyhemoglobin saturation (HbO$_2$) of single red blood cells within
tumor microvessels was determined.

Materials and methods

Inbred Sprague - Dawley rats of both sexes and anesthetized
with sodium - pentobarbital were used. The experimental tumors
were grown subcutaneously after injection of ascites cells of DS -
Carcinosarcoma into the dorsum of the left hind foot. Tumors were
used in experiments when they reached volumes ranging from 1.5 to
5.0 ml (10 to 17 days after implantation).

Local hyperthermia was induced by application of microwaves
(2.45 GHz), which were produced by a microwave generator and delivered through a special applicator. The power of the generator
was adjusted as required to hold the measured tumor temperature
constant to within 0.1°C. The temperature of the tumors was
monitored continuously with micro-thermocouples. The tissue sites
used for the monitoring of the mean temperature were not employed
for the measurement of the HbO$_2$ data. Thus, possible tissue
damage by the thermocouple did not affect the experimental results.
The core temperature of the animals was measured continually using
small thermistor probes. The core temperature did not change
substantially during microwave application to the hind foot dorsum.

In the present study three hyperthermia levels were employed:
40°C, 43°C, and 45°C. In all experiments the heat treatment lasted
for 30 minutes. In 10 unheated control tumors the mean tissue
temperature was approximately 35°C.

Monitoring of the mean arterial blood pressure and of the
relevant respiratory gas parameters was performed throughout all
experiments after cannulation of the carotid artery.

The oxyhemoglobin saturation of single red blood cells (HbO$_2$)
within tumor microvessels was studied utilizing a cyrophotometric
micromethod (12). After heating and subsequent normalization of
the tumor temperature, tissue biopsies were taken from the tumors
by means of special tongs which were precooled with liquid nitrogen.
The tissue biopsies were sectioned into 15/μm thin tissue slices
at -60°C. Afterwards HbO$_2$ data of single red blood cells were
measured at -100°C using a special ZEISS-photometer (for details
see 12, 13). Only HbO$_2$ data within microvessels having diameters
from 3 to 10 μm were included.

Results

    During control conditions (mean tissues temperature approx-
imately 35°C) the HbO$_2$ data obtained in tumors are scattered over
the whole saturation range from zero to 100 sat. %. The mean HbO$_2$
saturation value under these conditions is 51 sat. % (see fig. 1).
The median is 59 sat. %, the modal class being 65 - 70 sat. %.

    The cumulative frequency distribution curve of measured HbO$_2$
data in controls is shown in fig. 2, together with data obtained
immediately after heat treatment. From these curves there is clear
indication that upon heating at 40°C, the oxygenation of the tumor
tissue significantly improved (p<0.005). This is shown by a
distinct right-shift of the frequency distribution, i.e., a shift
to higher saturation values. Directly after 40°C hyperthermia, the
mean saturation increased to 66 sat. % (see fig. 1). The median
was 70 sat. %. Only 0.3% of the data obtained were on zero level.
At least 0.6% of the values were grouped into the lowest class.

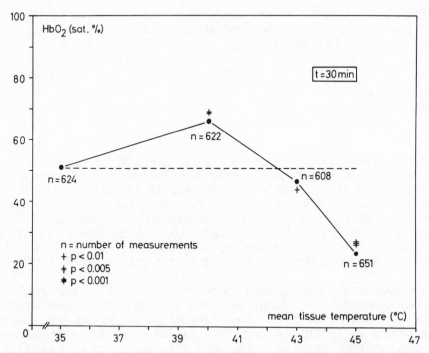

Figure 1. Mean HbO$_2$ data of single red blood cells within
tumor microvessels as a function of mean tumor temperature. Heat
application time: 30 minutes.

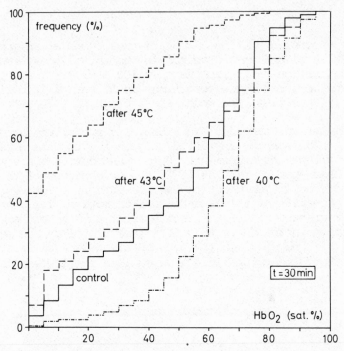

Figure 2.   Cumulative frequency distribution curves of HbO_2 data during control conditions and after localized heating for 30 minutes at 40°C, 43°C and 45°C.

In contradistinction to this, after 43°C hyperthermia, the tumor oxygenation significantly decreased as compared with control conditions ($p<0.01$).   At this hyperthermia level nearly 7% of the values were already grouped between zero and 5 sat. %.   After a further rise of the mean tumor temperature to 45°C, the tumor oxygenation drastically decreased ($p<0.001$).   Under these conditions approximately 4% of the measured HbO_2 values were on zero level. 24% of the data were grouped into the lowest saturation class.

Throughout all experiments no systemic effects of the host could be detected.   Therefore, systemic changes did not mask or enhance alterations in tumor blood flow or in the tissue oxygenation status caused by local hyperthermia.   In addition, all tumor biopsies were taken at comparable data for mean arterial blood pressure (140-144 mmHg), and for respiratory gas parameters in the arterial blood. For this reason and considering comparable mean tumor volumes in the

different hyperthermia groups, the results exclusively reflected
changes caused only by localized hyperthermia within the tumor
tissue itself.

Discussion

The present observations clearly suggest that local hyperthermia has profound effects on tumor tissue oxygenation. Experimental evidence has been obtained by measuring the oxyhemoglobin
saturation of single red blood cells within tumor microvessels.

Moderate hyperthermia ($40^{\circ}C$) led to an improvement of the
tumor tissue oxygenation as compared to physiological control
conditions. Temperatures higher that $42^{\circ}C$ resulted in decreasing
HbO_2 saturations. A 30 minute period of hyperthermia at $45^{\circ}C$ was
followed by a drastic fall of the HbO_2 values, progressing to very
low saturations. These findings are in agreement with recent
results showing that localized hyperthermia caused on the average
an improvement in the tissue oxygenation of C3H mouse mammary
adenocarcinoma at mean temperatures progressing to $40^{\circ}C$ (7). When
tissue temperatures exceeded this "temperature   optimum", a
distinct decline of the mean tissue pO_2 values became obvious,
both in small rodent tumors (7) and in human tumors (9).

The changes in the tumor oxygenation during hyperthermia seem
to be predominantly mediated through changes in tumor blood flow
(TBF), which showed the same directional changes (7). In those
experiments moderate hyperthermia ($39 - 41^{\circ}C$) increased TBF, whereas
temperatures higher than $42^{\circ}C$ were followed by a decline in TBF.
At $45^{\circ}C$ an almost complete cessation of nutritive blood flow
occurred due to a shutdown of microcirculation (7).

The flow improvement at already modest temperatures is most
likely caused by a dilatation of small blood vessels (11). This
dilatation is consistent with the observed "revival" of tumor
blood flow (8). No vessel damage is obvious at this hyperthermia
level (11). At intermediate temperatures ($42 - 43^{\circ}C$) marked
congestion and dilatation progressing to a severe and irreversible
vessel damage can be observed (11). These alterations are accompanied by stasis, extravasation of blood from vessels, microthrombosis and sludging of red blood cells. After $45^{\circ}C$-
hyperthermia, severe stasis, pronounced clotting and marked
hemorrhage are responsible for the almost complete shutdown of the
microcirculation. These changes occur along with the plugging of
tumor microvessels by rigid red blood cells due to severe tissue
acidosis.

Since the tumor biopsies were taken immediately after the tumor
temperature had reached control conditions, the HbO_2 distribution
cannot be affected by temperature changes on whole blood oxygen

affinity. However, during 45°C- hyperthermia, intensified tissue
acidosis, which has been described recently (7), leads to a right-
shift of the O_2 dissociation curve and, thus, supports the lowering
of the HbO_2 values of single red blood cells within tumor microvessels.

Considering the impact of eleveated temperatures on the O_2
consumption by the tumor cells (14), metabolic effects seem to have
minor influence on the HbO_2 distribution. This has been discussed
in detail in a preceding paper (8).

The results presented here are valid only for the time-temper-
ature combinations employed in this study. Increasing the heating
time up to 60 minutes, deteriorations of the microcirculation and
thus of the tumor oxygenation already occurred at modest hyperthermia
(40°C). This point is under investigation in our laboratory. The
extent of the microenvironmental alterations and the direction of
the variations, therefore, can be modified by variations of the
tissue temperature level and/or by the heat application time.

Blood flowing through a tissue influences the tissue temperature
distribution and vice versa. Therefore, when heating tumors one
is confronted with a crucial problem: The effectiveness of hyperthermia is unfortunately limited due to an inhomogeneous microflow
distribution and, hence, to a heterogeneous temperature field within
the tumor tissue. From this point of view, great intra-individual
and inter-individual differences in the response of the cellular
microenvironment to hyperthermia have to be expected. Pilot studies
in our laboratories concerning the temperature distribution within
the unheated tumors revealed considerable variations up to 1.5°C.

Summary

Upon heating at 40°C for 30 minutes, the oxygenation of the
tumor tissue significantly improved as compared with control conditions at 35°C. In contradistinction to this, the tumor oxygenation significantly decreased directly after 43°C- hyperthermia.
A further temperature rise to 45°C caused the oxygenation to drastically drop due to an almost complete cessation of nutritive blood
flow. The changes in tumor oxygenation during hyperthermia seem to
be predominantly mediated through changes in tumor blood flow, which
showed the same directional changes.

References

1. Dickson, J. A., The effects of hyperthermia in animal tumor
      systems. Rec. Res. Cancer Res. 59, 43, 1977.
2. Overgaard, J., Effect of hyperthermia on malignant cells in
      vivo. Cancer 39, 2637, 1977.
3. Suit, H. D., Hyperthermic effects on animal tissues. Radio-

logy 123, 483, 1977.

4. Gerweck, L. E., Nygaard, T. G., Burlett, M., Response of cells to hyperthermia under acute and chronic hypoxic conditions. Cancer Res. 39, 966, 1979.

5. Overgaard, J., Effect of hyperthermia on the hypoxic fraction in an experimental mammary carcinoma in vivo. Brit. J. Cancer 54, 245, 1981.

6. Gerweck, L. E., Richards, B., Influence of pH on the thermal sensitivity of cultured human glioblastoma cells. Cancer Res. 41, 845, 1981.

7. Vaupel, P., Frinak, S., Müller-Klieser, W., Bicher, H. I., Impact of localized hyperthermia on the cellular micro-environment in solid tumors. J. Nat. Cancer Inst. Mono. 60, in press, 1981.

8. Vaupel, P., Ostheimer, K., Müller-Klieser, W., Circulatory and metabolic responses of malignant tumors during localized hyperthermia. J. Cancer Res. Clin. Oncol. 98, 15, 1980.

9. Bicher, H. I., Hetzel, F. W., Sandhu, T. S., Frinak, S., Vaupel, P., O'Hara, M. D., O'Brien, T., Effects of hyperthermia on normal and tumor microenvironment. Radiology 137, 523, 1980.

10. Eddy, H. A., Alterations in tumor microvasculature during hyperthermia. Radiology 137, 515, 1980.

11. Emami, B., Nussbaum, G. H., Hahn, N., Piro, A. J., Dritschilo, A., Quimby, F., Histopathological study on the effect of hyperthermia on microvasculature. Int. J. Radiat. Oncol. Biol. Phys. 7, 343, 1981.

12. Grunewald, W. A., Lübbers, D. W., Kryophotometry as a method for analyzing the intracapillary HbO$_2$ saturation of organs under different O$_2$ supply conditions. Adv. exp. Med. Biol. 75, 55, 1976.

13. Vaupel, P., Manz, R., Müller-Klieser, W., Grunewald, W. A., Intracapillary HbO$_2$ saturation in malignant tumors during normoxia and hyperoxia. Microvasc. Res. 17, 181, 1979.

14. Muller-Klieser, W., Zander, R., Vaupel, P., Oxygen consumption of tumor cells suspended in native ascitic fluid at 1-42°C. Pflügers Arch. 377, R 17, 1978.

CARDIOVASCULAR AND OXYGENATION CHANGES

DURING WHOLE BODY HYPERTHERMIA

N.S. Faithfull, A.P. Van Den Berg, and
G.C. Van Rhoon

Erasmus University, Rotterdam, and
Rotterdam Radiotherapeutic Institute

Introduction

In the last few years, many reports of whole body hyperthermia treatment have appeared in literature. In most centres this is conducted under general anaesthesia, (1-6) others use a generalised sedation technique. (7-9) In depth studies of cardiovascular changes have been very few and far between and only two centres appear to have measured the cardiac output and pulmonary artery pressures. (4, 7) To date we have only found one group of investigators who have reported measurements of oxygen comsumption. (13)

In this paper we intend to demonstrate the major changes in the cardiovascular system. We will also discuss changes in oxygen consumption and oxygen availability in our patients. Finally we will report some results obtained by monitoring the oxygen saturation in hepatic venous blood.

Material and methods

The report concerns 25 treatments carried out under general anaesthesia. The patients were anaesthetised with a muscle relaxant, nitrous oxide, oxygen technique and were mechanically ventilated. They were heated using a modified Siemens technique. After placement on a warm water circulation mattress the patient is anaesthetised and the whole of the body apart from the head is covered in plastic film to prevent evaporation of sweat. The cabin is then closed. A body temperature of 41.8°C is reached in about one and a half hours and the patients are maintained at this plateau temperature for 2 hours. After opening the cabin and removal of the plastic film the patients cool rapidly.

Before, or in some cases after, the induction of anaesthesia
the following intravascular lines were inserted: an intra arterial
cathether was inserted into the radial artery at the wrist for
arterial pressure monitoring and arterial blood gas and acid base
estimations; a Swan Ganz catheter was inserted into the left sub-
clavian vein and advanced into the pulmonary artery. Through this
catheter we could measure pulmonary artery pressures, pulmonary
capillary wedge pressures and, by means of a thermodilution
technique, cardiac output. A catheter was inserted into the femoral
vein in the inguinal region and advanced under an image intensifier
into one of the hepatic veins. Its position was confirmed radio-
graphically before and after warming the patient. Through this
catheter the central venuous pressure was monitored and the hepatic
venous blood was sampled.

Results

In Table 1 the cardiovascular haemodynamics of the systemic
circulation is shown. The most important of these results are
displayed graphically in figure 1. In Table 2 the changes in the
pulmonary circulation are tabulated and some of these, together
with the cardiac index, are displayed in figure 2.

As far as the systemic side of the circulation is concerned,
the work performed by the ventricle, though increased at the beginning of plateau, is significantly decreased at mid plateau and at
that time it is not significantly different from values obtained
in the awake patients. These patients were premedicatied with
papaveratum and hyoscine and in some cases had also received
intravenous diazepam while intravascular monitoring lines were
inserted. This decrease in left ventricular work index, is caused
by a significant fall of mean arterial pressure in the presence of
slowly declining systemic vascular resistance index. Due to large
reductions in systemic vascular resistance taking place during
warming, the left ventricular work is never proportionally so
increased as the cardiac index. An interesting and constant finding
is a significant decrease of mean arterial pressure at 15 minutes of
cooling followed by a very significant rise at 30 minutes of cooling.

When looking at the right ventricular work index we see that
it is proportionately increased far above the increase in left
ventricular work index, which increases 120% between the beginning
and end of warming. On the other hand the right ventricular work
increases by 260%. This appears not to be due to a proportionally
lesser decrease of peripheral resistance in the pulmonary circulation
than occurs in the systemic circulation but by the presence of a
significantly raised mean pulmonary artery pressure.

Figure 3 represents graphically the changes brought about by
WBHT on cardiac index, haemoglobin content of the blood and oxygen

Table 1 The effects of Whole Body Hyperthemia (2 hrs. at 41.8°C) on the systemic circulation. Means + 1sem. Significance is indicated using the Paired t test in comparison with the previous data point P <.05 - x, P <.01 = xx, P <.001 = xxx.

| | Before Anesthesia | Before Warming | Plateau Temperature 41.8°C | | | After 15 min cooling T°=40,7°C ± 0,1 | After 30 min cooling T°=39,6°C ± 0,1 | After 45 min cooling T°=38,9°C ± 0,2 |
			Beginning	mid	end			
Mean Arterial Pressure (mm Hg)	82,8 + 3,1	76,8 + 2,8	71,9 + 2,8 ***	62,3 + 1,9 *	62,6 + 1,9	58,1 + 2,4 *	63,6 + 2,1 **	66,8 + 3,0
Heart Rate (beats min^{-1})	97 + 4	84 + 3	126 + 4 ***	143 + 5 ***	145 + 4	141 + 5	136 + 4	135 + 5
Cardiac Index (L $min^{-1}\ m^{-2}$)	4,2 + 0,4	3,3 + 0,4 *	7,6 + 0,5 ***	7,0 + 0,4	7,6 + 0,4	6,7 + 0,5	6,7 + 0,3	6,4 + 0,5 *
Pulmonary Capillary Wedge Pressure (mm Hg)	5,9 + 1,2	8,3 + 0,8 *	8,4 + 0,7	8,0 + 0,8	8,1 + 0,6	9,3 + 0,6	10,2 + 0,8	9,0 + 0,5
Left Ventricular Work Index (Kgm m min^{-1})	4,6 + 0,5	3,1 + 0,3 *	7,0 + 0,6 ***	5,3 + 0,4 **	5,7 + 0,4	4,8 + 0,7	4,7 + 0,3	5,3 + 0,6 *
Systemic Vascular Resistance Index (Dynes sec cm^{-5})	1585 + 112	1966 + 207 *	743 + 60 ***	659 + 64	603 + 42	624 + 50	624 + 38	722 + 56

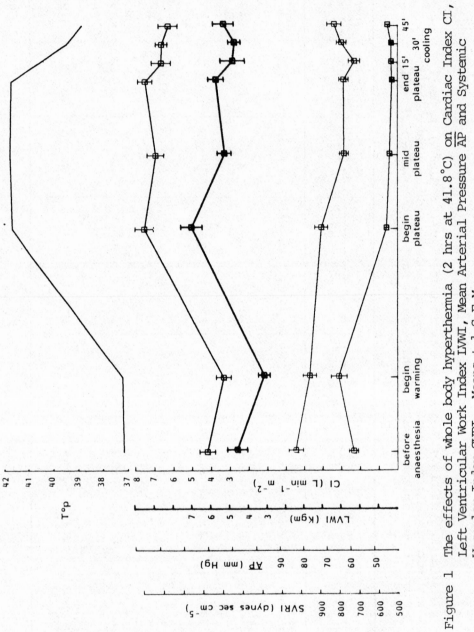

Figure 1   The effects of whole body hyperthermia (2 hrs at 41.8°C) on Cardiac Index CI, Left Ventricular Work Index LVWI, Mean Arterial Pressure $\overline{AP}$ and Systemic Vascular Index SVRI. Means ± 1 S.E.M.

Table 2 The effects of Whole Body Hyperthermia (2 hrs. at 41.8°C) on the pulmonary circulation. Means + 1sem. Significance is indicated using the paired t test in comparison with the previous data point. P <0.5 = x, P <.01 = xx, P <.001 = xxx.

| | Before Anesthesia | Before Warming | Plateau Temperature 41.8°C | | | After 15 min cooling T°=40,7°C ± 0,1 | After 30 min cooling T°=39,6°C ± 0,1 | After 45 min cooling T°=38,9°C ± 0,2 |
			Beginning	mid	end			
Mean Pulmonary Artery Pressure (mm Hg)	13,9 + 1,4	13,6 + 1,0	15,5 + 1,0 **	14,5 + 1,13	14,6 + 1,1	15,6 + 1,4	16,5 + 1,3	15,5 + 1,8
Central Venous Pressure (mm Hg)	1,0 + 2,0	5,3 + 2,1	5,5 + 1,7	5,0 + 1,6	5,4 + 1,7	5,2 + 1,4	8,3 + 0,9	8,0 + 0,0
Right Ventricular Work Index (Kgm m min^{-1})	0,47 + 0,10	0,25 + 0,04 *	0,96 + 0,12 **	0,76 + 0,17	0,82 + 0,14	0,48 + 0,14	0,81 + 0,16	0,76 + 0,00
Pulmonary Vascular Resistance Index (Dynes sec cm^{-5})	262 + 41	240 + 40	120 + 12 *	100 + 17	104 + 25	130 + 40	136 + 36	94 + 0

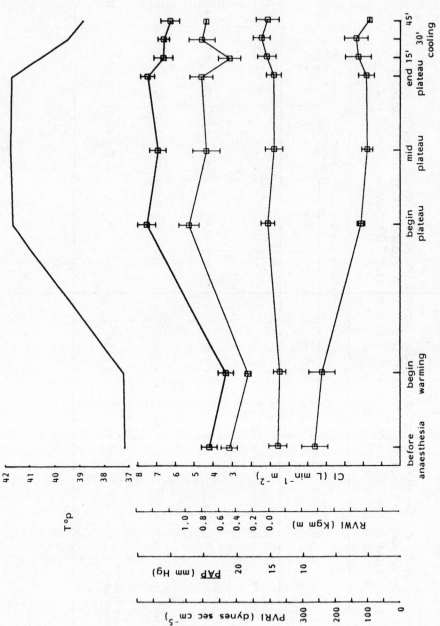

Figure 2   The effects of whole body hyperthermia (2 hrs at 41.8°C) on Cardiac Index CI, Right Ventricular Work Index RVWI, Mean Pulmonary Arterial Pressure $\overline{PAP}$ and Pulmonary Vascular Resistance Index PVRI. Means ± 1 S.E.M.

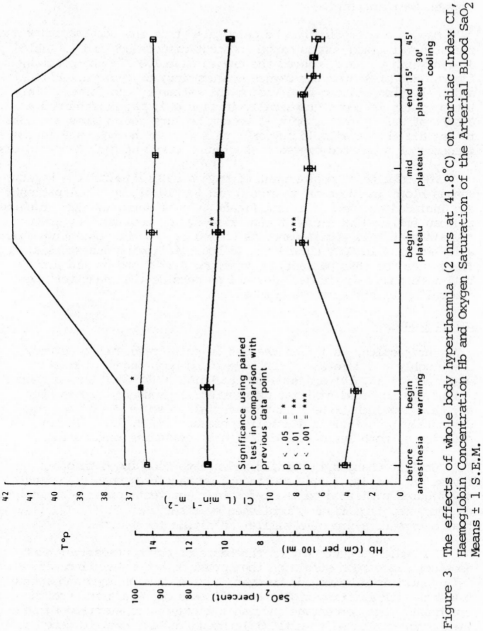

Figure 3 The effects of whole body hyperthermia (2 hrs at 41.8°C) on Cardiac Index CI, Haemoglobin Concentration Hb and Oxygen Saturation of the Arterial Blood SaO$_2$ Means ± 1 S.E.M.

saturation of the arterial blood (corrected for temperature). All three factors are intimately concerned with the transport of oxygen from the lungs to the tissues which is often loosely referred to as "oxygen availability".

Oxygen consumption can be calculated from the cardiac index and the arterial mixed venous oxygen content differences and in Table 3, (in which we have ignored the oxygen dissolved in the plasma), figures are presented for oxygen consumption, oxygen availability, and the ratio obtained by dividing the latter by the former. This ratio, which is shown graphically in figure 4, may be regarded as a sort of safety factor only if we can be sure the tissues are able to use all the "available oxygen"; this may not be the case in the presence of a shifted oxygen dissociation curve at high temperatures.

The results of measurement of oxygen saturation in the hepatic venous blood is shown in figures 5 and 6. In figure 5 all patients are included and we see a significant fall of saturation on reaching plateau followed by a significant rise during cooling. Figure 6 reveals that this significance is caused by the one patient who had a marked rise in SGOT during the 48 hours following anaesthesia. The values for this patient, on reaching 41.8°C and at mid plateau, fall more than two standard deviations outside the means for the "normal" patients at those points.

Discussion

Our results, as far as changes in pulse rate are concerned, are roughly the same as others have found both under general anaesthesia, (5, 10) and sedation techniques (7, 9). Some authors, (7) have also found similiar mean arterial pressure changes, but may have found that the fall in arterial pressure was caused predominately by a fall in diastolic pressure (8, 9, 11). In our experience, both systolic and diastolic pressures tend to fall.

Similar changes in cardiac index have been found in other investigations (4, 7, 14) and though we have been unable to find any figures published on the left and right ventricular work indices we conclude, from figures published by other authors (7, 12, 14), that our results are of a similar magnitude to theirs.

We would suggest that on the basis of our own results, WBHT does not place much strain on the normal or moderately incapacitated left ventricle. We would, however, advice caution when subjecting patients with existing right heart disease or strain to hyperthermia treatment. Our percentage increases in oxygen consumption agree with other published results (13) though we have not, to date, seen details of oxygen transport calculations. From our own observations we would conclude that there should be no problem in delivery of oxygen to the tissues under WBHT.

Table 3 The effects of Whole Body Hyperthermia (2 hrs. at 41.8°C) on oxygen consumption, oxygen 'availability' and the ratio between the two. Means + 1 sem. Significance is indicated using the paired t test in comparison with the previous data point P <.05 = x, P <.01 = xx, P <.001 = xxx.

	Before Anesthesia	Before Warming	Plateau Temperature 41.8°C			After 30 min cooling T°=39,6°C +0,1
			Beginning	mid	end	
Oxygen Consumption (ml min⁻¹ m⁻²)	97 + 8	101 + 14	138 + 13 **	140 + 10		121 + 9 *
Oxygen Availability (ml min⁻¹ m⁻²)	502 + 40	514 + 89	1068 + 75 **	978 + 55		900 + 67
Ratio Oxygen Availability/Oxygen Consumption	5,18 + 0,37	5,04 + 0,37	7,94 + 0,42 **	7,43 + 0,35		7,49 + 0,40

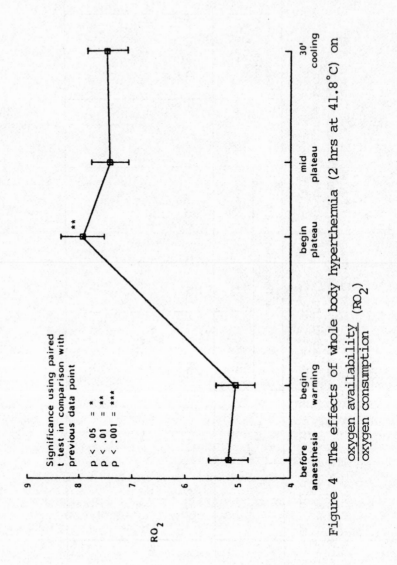

Figure 4   The effects of whole body hyperthermia (2 hrs at 41.8°C) on

$$\frac{\text{oxygen availability}}{\text{oxygen consumption}} \quad (RO_2)$$

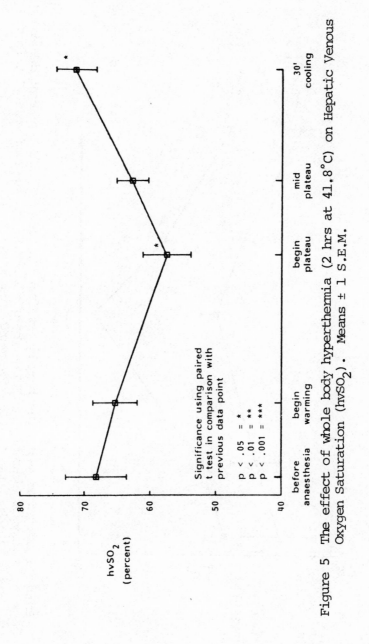

Figure 5 The effect of whole body hyperthermia (2 hrs at 41.8°C) on Hepatic Venous Oxygen Saturation (hvSO$_2$). Means ± 1 S.E.M.

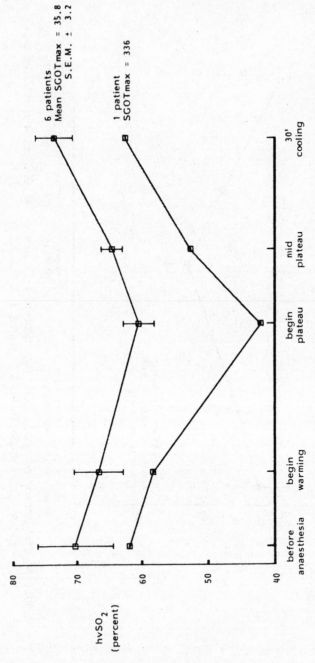

Figure 6   The effects of whole body hyperthermia (2 hrs at 41.8°C) on Hepatic Venous Oxygen Saturation (hvSO$_2$). Means ± 1 S.E.M. and the maximum SGOT values in the first 48 hours following treatment.

As far as we know there are no published data of hepatic venous oxygen saturations under hyperthermia. From our very limited experience we would suggest that this measurement may have prognastic value with regard to post hyperthermia liver damage.

Acknowledgement

This research is supported by the Koningin Wilhelmina Funds, Grant No. EUR 7704.

References

1. Pettigrew, R. T., Cancer therapy by whole body heating. Int. Proc. of the Int. Symposium on Cancer Therapy by Hyperthermia and Radiation, Washington D.C., p 282-288, Arpil, 1975.
2. Blair, R. M., and Levin. W., Clinical experience of the induction and maintanence of whole body hyperthermia. Proc. of the 2nd Int. Symposium on Cancer Therapy by Hyperthermia and Radiation, Essen, p. 318-321, 1977.
3. MacKenzie, A., McLeod, K., Cassels-Smith, A. J., Dickson, J. A. Total body hyperthermia: Techniques and patient management. Proc. Int. Symposium on Cancer Therapy by Hyperthermia and Radiation, Washington D. C., p. 272-282, 1975.
4. Parks, L. C., Minaberry D, Smith, D. P., Neeley, W. A. Treatment of far-advanced bronchogenic carcinoma by extracorporeally induced systemic hyperthermia. J. Thoracic Cardiovasc. Surg. 78, p 883- 392, 1979.
5. Barlogie, P. M., Corry, P. M., Yip, E., Lippman, L., Johnston, D. A., Khalil, K., Tenczyncki, T. F., Reilly, E., Lawson, R., Doisik, G., Rigor, B., Hankenson, R., and Freireich, E. J. Total-body hyperthermia with and without chemotherapy for advanced human neoplasms. Cancer Research, 39, p 1481-1489, May, 1979.
6. Euler-Rolle, J., Priesching, A., Vormittag, E., Tschakaloff, C., Polterauer, P. Prevention of cardiac complications during whole-body hyperthermia by beta receptor blockage. Proc. of the 2nd Int. Symposium on Cancer Therapy by Hyperthermia and Radiation, Essen, p 302-305, 1977.
7. Lees, D. E., Young, D. K., Bull, J. M., Whang-Peng, J., Schuette, W., Smith, R. N., Macnarmara, T. E. Anaesthetic Management of Whole Body Hyperthermia for the Treatment of Cancer, Anesthesiology, 52, p 418-428, 1980.
8. Logawney-Malik, Bhalla, Thomas. Effects of Hyperthermia on renal functions, Ind. J. Med. Res., 69, pp 312-318, 1979.
9. Ostrow, S., Echo Van, D., Whitacre, M., Aisner, J., Simon, R., Wiernik, P. H. Physiologic response and toxicity in patients undergoing whole body hyperthermia for the treatment of cancer. Cancer Treatment Reports, 65, p 323-325, 1981.

10. Pettigrew, R. T., Galt, J. M., Ludgate, C. M., Horn, D. B.,
    Smith, A. N. Circulatory and biochemical effects of
    whole body hyperthermia. Brit. J. Surg. 61, p 727-730,
    1974.
11. Larkin, J. M., Sterling Edwards, W., Smith, D. E., Clark, P. J.
    Systemic thermotherapy: Description of a method and
    physiologic tolerance in clinical subjects. Cancer, 40,
    p 3155-3159, 1977.
12. Kim, Y. D., Lees, D. E., Bull, J., Whang-Peng, J., Schuette, W.,
    MacNamara, T. Hyperthermic Potentiation of the alpha-
    adrenergic blockade induced by droperidol. A. S. A.
    Congress, 1978.
13. Lees, D. E., Young, D. K., Schuette, W., Bull, J., Whang-Peng,
    J. Causes of induced hyperthermia. Anaesthesiology, 50
    p 69-70.
14. Young, K. D., Lake, C. R., Lees, D. E., Schuette, W. H., Bull,
    J. M., Weise, V., Kopin, I. J. Hemodynamic and plasma
    catecholamine responses to hyperthermia cancer therapy
    in humans. Am. J. Physiol., 237(5), p H570-H574.

RECENT TRENDS IN THE CANCER MULTISTEP THERAPY CONCEPT

Manfred von Ardenne and Winfried Krüger

Research Institute Manfred von Ardenne, 8051 Dresden,
Zeppelinstrabe 7, G. D. R.

Introduction

It is a commonplace that the cure rates of most types of cancer
are far from total: surgical removal of tumors is often necessarily
incomplete, all of the antitumor drugs have side effects, and
irradiation includes several hazards and injuries as well.

In order to reduce inherent disadvantages and to improve
therapeutic results these three measures have been combined jointly
for decades. Thus, the idea of linking different steps in fighting
against cancer is well known to all oncologists. Taken altogether,
however, the state of the art is entirely unsatisfactory despite
the progress achieved with these classical weapons.

No wonder that hyperthermia has seen a notable renaissance in
search of a way out of this dilemma. However, hyperthermia cannot
be expected to be the only clue to all problems unsolved in cancer
therapy. Hyperthermia will never replace surgery, but in cases of
surgical inaccessibility of certain tumors this modality could
become a true alternative and, moreover, a valuable adjunct or
supplement to present radio- and chemotherapy. Multiple attempts
for combining hyperthermia with radiation or drugs point to this
direction (1).

One of the primary goals of cancer research is to define
differences between normal and neoplastic cells that can be used as
a point of attack in tumor therapy. Even if no qualitative differences exist, quantitative differences may be large enough to serve
the same purpose. They represent the rationale of any combination
therapy.

With this in mind, we remembered the early findings by Otto Warburg (2) that an elevated rate of glycolysis is one of the most consistent biochemical characteristics of tumor cells, as well as the paper by Voegtlin, Fitch, Kahler et al. (3) Reporting a pH drop in experimental tumors after parenteral administration of glucose. We rendered these general findings therapeutically utilizable by introducing systemic long-term glucose infusion up to the five-fold of the normal, which causes a pH drop in the order of 1 pH unit in tumors (4). On combining this tumor hyperacidi-fication with hyperthermia we found as early as in 1968 that low pH and high temperature act synergistically on tumor cell killing in vitro (5) as is shown in Figure 1. This effect has been confirmed repeatedly by others (6, 7, 8, 9) and discussed under several aspects (10, 11, 12). Further investigations centered the effect of low pH and/or hyperthermia on lysosomes (13) and on vascular functions in neoplastic tissues (14, 15).

Since the early days of our Cancer Multistep Therapy (CMT) research (16) hyperthermia and tumor overacidification represent constantly its two fundamentals. The concept itself has been necessarily subject to several modifications, concerning number, type and timing of additional attacks. Results obtained from experiments and preliminary clinical trials elucidated the prominent role of the tumor microenvironment (microcirculation and substrate supply) as the main target of hyperthermia and low pH under in vitro conditions (17, 18, 19).

The Capillary Bed of Tumors as a Main Target of the CMT

Figure 2 demonstrates the changes occurring in a capillary vessel during normo- and hyperthermia, as was measured by Dr. Ernest using vital microscopy (unpublished results). Initially, the blood flow increases with increasing temperature as was observed also by Vaupel et al (20) using different methods. At temper-atures over 40°C the blood flow begins to decrease and reaches its minimum at temperatures around 42°C due to the disappearance of the plasma border and increased interactions between blood cells and the inner vessel wall. The swelling of the vessel wall at elevated temperatures is not yet considered here, although this effect contributes to the blood flow stagnation as well. This diagram confirms the well-known fact that with respect to blood flow temperatures around 41°C are not yet critical for normal tissues. However, in tumors hyperacidified by systemic long-term glucose infusion these processes proceed more rapidly. The low pH in the interstitium reacts upon the red cells in the venules and diminishes their flexibility (20, 21). Moreover, leukocytes become more sticky and promote the vascular occlusion. Under convenient conditions, i.e., acidification before hyperthermia, the capillary obstruction is complete and irreversible selectively in tumor tissues (21). The multifactorial process of vascular obstruction is summarized

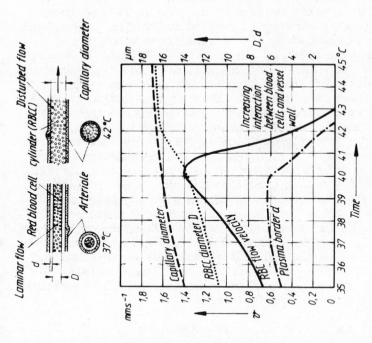

Figure 2 – Dependency of vascular and rheological parameters in capillaries on temperature,
obtained by Dr. Ernest Dresden from vitalmicro-
scopic measurements.

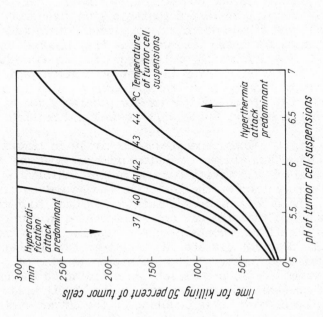

Figure 1 – Amplification of the thermal
sensitivity of Ehrlich ascites carcinoma
cells at pH values below 7.0 adjusted with
lactic acid in vitro. Simulation of in vivo
conditions: percentage of suspending cells:
0.5; glucose concentration 1 mg/100 mL;
percentage of oxygen in the gas phase: 0.3
(7).

in Figure 3. The mechanism shown here was proposed first at the
Hyperthermia Conference in Essen, West Germany, in 1977, and was
quoted by others at the Fort Collins Conference in 1979 so that it
can be thought a proposal worthy to be discussed. The present form
was modified with consideration of the results obtained by Dr.
Ernest in Dresden. The chart of the next slide (Figure 4) shows
how we imagine the cooperative effects of low pH and high temperature
on the microcirculation in tumor tissues and how these factors
initiate finally tumor cell killing. This representation is based
on own results as well as on those obtained by other authors. I
am referring for example to Holger Schmid-Schönbein, Aachen, his
brother Geert S.-S., formerly at Columbia University, New York,
presently in California, and A. L. Copley, Polytechnic Institute,
Brooklyn, N.Y. The scheme shown here does not fully consider all
the interrelationships and interactions and should be seen not so
much as an elaborated concept rather than a starting point for
further discussion. Nevertheless, we are convinced that the
selective element for tumor cell killing comes from the combination
of heat and low pH. The generation of systemic high glucose levels
for stimulation tumor cell glycolysis is now well established and
its applicability for patients was proven in clinical trials. Let
me turn now to the second point of my presentation: the generation
of adequately high temperatures in tumors.

Hyperthermia Using the CMT Selectotherm Technique

     According to Jain (22) the temperature field in a tissue is
determined by heat conduction and convection, metabolic heat
generation, thermal energy transferred to the tissue from an
external source, and the tissue geometry. The most common mathematical representation for these parameters is the "bio-heat
transfer equation". The discussion of this equation reveals that
reduced blood flow and elevated metabolic heat generation facilitate
the further temperature rise by heat transfer from outside into a
tumor of given geometry. These conditions are precisely met by
the CMT Selectotherm technique, which will be outlined briefly now.

     Firstly, the low pH values generated selectively in tumors by
means of systemic long-term glucose infusion into the host are the
most effective source of selectivity because of its inhibiting
influence on microcirculation of the target tissue as was outlined
before. Secondly, the excess glucose itself contributes to metabolic
heat generation provided that the patient is breathing synchronously
an oxygen-enriched air mixture containing 40% oxygen. As is known
excess glucose alone does not elevate the core temperature, but the
glucose-oxygen combination does. This combination is also of
advantage to all normal cells, stabilizes the circulation and makes
any application of anesthetics unneccessary during hyperthermic
treatment. On the other hand, this doubling of the oxygen content
of the inspiration air does not yet influence the oxygen supply of

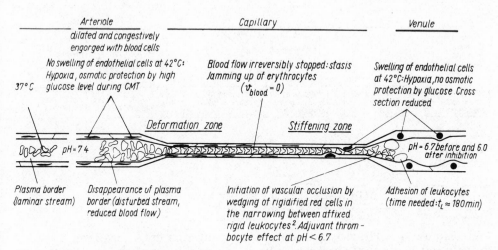

Figure 3 - Conception of the mechanism of vascular occlusion in the capillary-postcapillary bed (hemostasis, microthrombosis by combining optimized tumor tissue hyperacidification (pH = 6.0) with local hyperthermia at 42.5°C (CMT Selectotherm technique), possibly combined with short-term blood pressure reduction. (1) 1977/80 CMT concept.

Primary effect: Structural rearrangement of all biomembranes involved at the transition site capillary/venule (rigidifying of red and white cells at pH decrease from 7.4 to <6.7)

1. Short-term blood flow inhibition, e.g., by local or systemic reduction of the propulsing blood pressure, promotes initiation of vascular obstruction (reduced shear rate diminishes blood fluidity).

2. Rich in lysosomes; discharge and activation of lysosomal enzymes at low pH: additional contribution to stiffening of blood cells. Further: accumulation of platelets and fibrin deposits in the proximate parts of the venules.

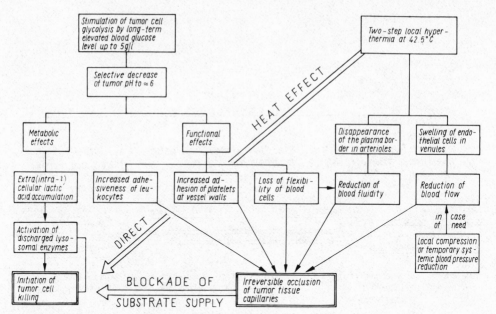

Figure 4 – Rheological and functional elements involved in triggering hemostasis selectively in tumor tissues during the Cancer Multistep Therapy process.

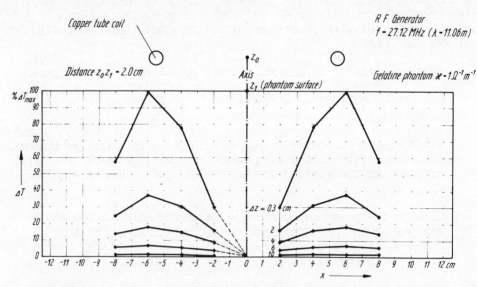

Figure 5 – Temperature profiles expressed as ΔT (percentage of T_{max}) in different depths of a gelatine phantom during eddy-current heating by the rf magnetic field of a ring coil ($r = 5.5$ cm). Large temperature inhomogeneities and marked temperature drop with increased depth (27).

solid tumors as was described by Vaupel and coworkers (23). A
metabolic shift in the tumor area from glycolysis to respiration
which would result in decreased lactic acid production is therefore
not to be feared. Instead of this, a core temperature elevation
in the range of 1.0 to 1.5°C can be observed regularly (24). A
core temperature of 38 or 38.5°C is, of course, too low for tumor
treatment, but represents a convenient starting point for further
temperature elevation by means of an external source. Hyperthermia
proper is generated by classical radiofrequency with 27.12 MHz,
however using a movable ring coil. Our preceding experiments had
shown that the temperature distribution is very inhomogeneous in a
gelatin phantom by using a fixed applicator coil. This is shown in
Figure 5. The temperature peaked expectedly at the surface of the
phantom directly below the coil and decreased rapidly with increasing
depth. However, when the rf source is shifted perpetually parallel
to the phantom surface, the temperature distribution becomes more
homogeneous in a larger area (Figure 6). The most important
practical effect of a scanning motion like this is that even in a
depth of 12 cm the temperature increase is still about 20% of the
maximum value. This basic principle of our CMT Selectotherm
technique, its mathematical modelling and physico-technical back-
ground were described in more detail in several papers (25, 26, 27,
28, 29). Figure 7 shows the experimental setting-up of the first
Selectotherm generation. The shield of the driving unit, which
controls the scanning motion, is removed here. As was already
mentioned, the practical hyperthermic treatment of patients is
performed in two steps (Figure 8). Firstly, the core temperature
is elevated to 41°C by scanning the trunk with high amplitudes in
x and y direction parallel to the body's surface. Secondly, the
amplitude of the rf source is reduced and focussed on the tumor
area. If necessary, also the draining lymph nodes can be heated
locally in a third step, so that in principle a "fractionated total
body hyperthermia" at 42.5°C can be performed, avoiding the known
risks occurring at one-step total hyperthermia at this temperature.

The course of temperature during a clinical trial is shown
in Figure 9. The initial rectal temperature indicates the contribution of the metabolic heat generation stimulated by excess
glucose and inhalation of oxygen-enriched air. In this case, where
an inoperable lung carcinoma was treated, we were not yet able to
measure the tumor temperature directly. Therefore, measurement
was made in the right chest muscle 2.5 cm beneath the skin in order
to obtain at least a guiding value. Further studies including
intratumoral temperature measurements also in such difficult cases
are at present under way in order to confirm the desired temperature
levels also in deep-seated tumors. Figure 10 shown the application
of the CMT Selectotherm device in case of an inoperable sarcoma of
the knee.

It is necessary to add that clinical trials like these have

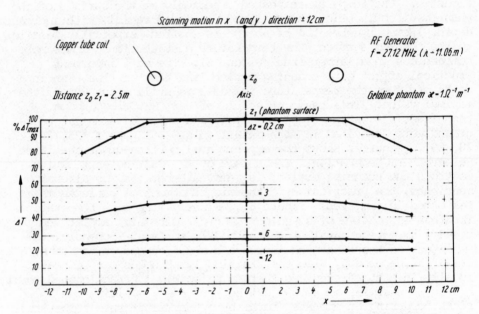

Figure 6 – Temperature profiles of a gelatine phantom (as in
figure 5), but using a scanning coil. Homogenized temperature
distribution and reduced temperature drop in the depth (27).

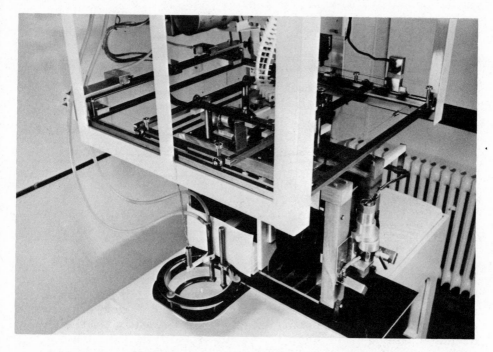

Figure 7 - Experimental applicator design of the first generation, working at 27.12 MHz and with water cooling; shields removed
(27).

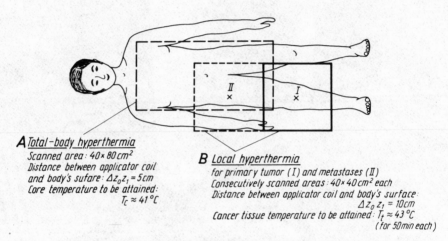

A <u>Total-body hyperthermia</u>
Scanned area: 40 × 80 cm²
Distance between applicator coil
and body's sufare: $\Delta z_0 z_1 = 5 cm$
Core temperature to be attained:
$T_c \approx 41 °C$

B <u>Local hyperthermia</u>
for primary tumor (I) and metastases (II)
Consecutively scanned areas: 40 × 40 cm² each
Distance between applicator coil and body's surface:
$\Delta z_0 z_1 = 10 cm$
Cancer tissue temperature to be attained: $T_t \approx 43 °C$
(for 50 min each)

Figure 8 – Principle of total body and local hyperthermia application using the CMT Selectotherm device. Parameters given are examples and can be modified at choice depending on the individual case.

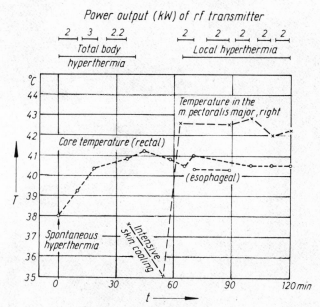

Figure 9 – Temperature courses during treatment of a patient suffering from an inoperable lung carcinoma with the CMT Seclecto-therm technique. Direct tumor temperature measurement was not possible for technical reasons. The temperature of the m. pectoralis major (2.5 cm beneath the skin surface) reflects, therefore, only approximately the true tumor temperature.

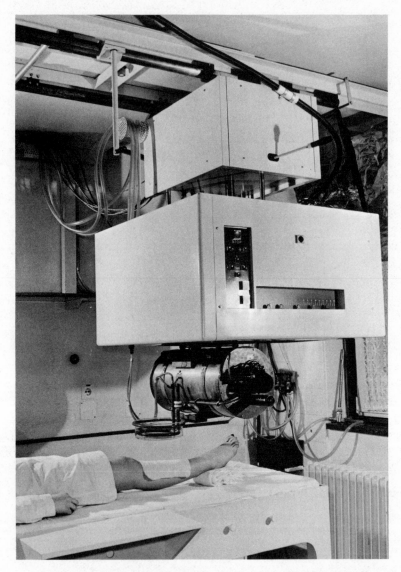

Figure 10 - Rf applicator of the second generation (CMT Selectotherm) for clinical trials (29).

been made in accord with all ethical standards internationally accepted and under the leadership of an experienced group of physicians. Our institute is neither a clinic nor a specified medical research institution, but a technical institute for research and development. Therefore, we are dependent on the cooperation with oncological clinics that are solely able to decide whether our conceptions are right or wrong.

Concluding Remarks

1. Low pH and high temperature fortify mutually in tumor destruction. Not only the malignant cells, but also the vascular system of the tumor including its constituents, such as blood cells, vessel walls, clotting factors, etc., are affected by this concerted action.

2. Therefore, hyperthermic treatment of tumors should be applied, if ever possible, in conjunction with optimum tumor acidification.

3. In order to avoid any risks for patients and to achieve sufficiently high temperatures in the target tissue, hyperthermia should be performed as a two-step procedure. Metabolic heat generation stimulated by excess glucose (for tumor acidification) plus oxygen (for stabilization of circulation) are concomitantly exploited for core temperature elevation. Target tissue temperatures of 42.5°C will be attained much easier in a preheated body ($\Delta T = 42.5^\circ - 41^\circ = 1.5^\circ$) than in a normothermic body ($\Delta T = 42.5^\circ C - 37^\circ = 5.5^\circ$).

4. The limitations of communly used radiofrequency heating can be overcome by the scanning principle. This principle results in homogenizing the temperature field in all three dimensions of the target.

5. The combined application of low pH and high temperature to tumors represents the ideal basic therapy and is open for additional attacks, such as pH-sensitive drugs, immunostimulants, irradiation etc.

References

1. Dethlefsen LA (ed.), The Third International Symposium: Cancer Therapy by Hyperthermia, Drugs and Radiation. Abstracts. Fort Collins, Co.: Colorado State Univ., June 22-26, 1980.
2. Warburg, O., The Metabolism of Tumors. London: Constable, 1930.
3. Voegtlin C., Fitch, R. H., Kahler, H., Johnson, J. M., Thompson, J. W., The influence of the parenteral administration of certain sugars on the pH of malignant tumors. Nat. Inst. Health Bull 164: 1, 1935.
4. von Ardenne, M., Reitnauer, P. G., Schmidt, D., Theoretische Grundlagen und in-vivo-Messungen zur Optimierung der selektiven Übersäuerung von Krebsgewebe. Acta Biol. Med. Germ 22: 35, 1969.
5. von Ardenne, M., Reitnauer, P. G., Selektive Krebszellen-schädigung durch Proteindenaturierung. Dtsch Gesundh-Wesen 23: 1681, 1968.
6. Freeman, M. L., Dewey, W. C., Hopwood, L. E., Effect of pH on hyperthermic cell survival. J. Natl. Cancer Inst. 58: 1837, 1977.
7. Gerweck, L. E., Modification of cell lethality at elevated temperatures. The pH effect. Radiation Res. 70: 224, 1977.
8. Gerweck, L. E., Jennings, M., Richards, B., Influence of pH on the response of cells to single and split doses of hyperthermia. Cancer Res. 40: 4019, 1980.
9. Gerweck, L, E., Richards, B., Influence of pH on the thermal sensitivity of cultured human glioblastoma cells. Cancer Res. 42: 845, 1981.
10. Overgaard, J., Influence of extracellular pH on the viability and morphology of tumor cell growth to hyperthermia. Cancer Res. 56: 1243, 1976.
11. Overgaard, J., Effect of hyperthermia on malignant cells in vivo. A review and a hypothesis. Cancer 39: 2637, 1977.
12. Overgaard, J. Nielsen, O. S., The role of tissue environmental factors on the kinetics and morphology of tumors exposed to hyperthermia. Ann NY Acad Sci. 335: 254, 1980.
13. von Ardenne, M., Krüger, W., Local tissue hyperacidification and lysosomes. In Dingle, J. T., Jacques, P. H., Shaw, I. H. (eds), Lysosomes in Applied Biology and Therapeutics. Vol. 6. Amsterdam: North Holland, Publ. Comp., 1977, p 161.
14. von Ardenne, M., Reitnauer, P. G., Selective occlusion of cancer tissue capillaries as central mechanism of Cancer Multistep Therapy. Jpn. J. Clin. Oncol. 10: 31, 1980.
15. Song, C. W., Effect of hyperthermia on vascular functions of normal tissue and experimental tumors. J. Natl. Cancer Inst. 60: 711, 1978.
16. von Ardenne, M., Theoretische und experimentelle Grundlagen der Krebs-Mehrschritt-Therapie. 2nd ed, Berlin: Volk and Gesundheit, 1970/71.

17. von Ardenne, M., Prinzipien und Konzept 1974 der Krebs-
    Mehrschritt-Therapie. Radio Biol., Radiother 16: 99, 1975.
18. von Ardenne, M., Prinzipien und Konzept 1977 der Krebs-
    Mehrschritt-Therapie. Arch Geschwulstforsch 48: 504, 1978.
19. von Ardenne, M., Über den Entwicklungsstand der Krebs-
    Mehrschritt-Therapie. Med. in uns Zeit 3: 34, 1979.
20. Vaupel, P., Ostheimer, K., Müller-Klieser, W. Circulatory and
    metabolic responses of malignant tumors during localized
    hyperthermia. J. Cancer Res. Clin. Oncol. 98: 15, 1980.
21. von Ardenne, M., Reitnauer, P. G., Gewebe-Übersäuerung und
    Mikrozirkulation. Arch Geschwulstforsch 48: 729, 1978.
22. Jain, R. K., Temperature distribution in normal and neoplastic
    tissues during normothermia and hyperthermia. Ann NY
    Acad. Sci. 335: 48, 1980.
23. Vaupel, P., Thews, G., Wendling, P., Kritische Sauerstoff-
    und Glucoseversorgung maligner Tumoren. Klin Wschr 101:
    1810, 1976.
24. von Ardenne, M., Vereinfachung der Krebs-Mehrschritt-Therapie
    durch induzierte Spontanhyperthermie. Krebsgeschehen 8:
    26, 1976.
25. von Ardenne, M., von Ardenne, T., Böhme, G., Dekawellen-
    Rasterhyperthermie. Ein neues Diathermieverfahren mit
    homogenisierter Energiezufuhr und sehr hoher Tiefenwirkung
    in Körpergewebe. Z Physiother 29: 225, 1977.
26. von Ardenne, M., On a new physical principle for selective
    local hyperthermia. in Streffer C. (ed); Cancer Therapy
    by Hyperthermia and Radiation. Baltimore-Munich, Urban
    and Schwarzenberg, 1978, p 96.
27. von Ardenne, M., Böhme, G., Kell, E., Reitnauer, P. G., Die
    Bedeutung der Warmeleitung für die therapeutischen
    Grenzen der selektiven Lokalhyperthermie von Krebsgeweben.
    Arch Geschwulstforsch, 47: 487, 1977.
28. von Ardenne, M., Bohme, G., Kell, E., On the optimization of
    local hyperthermy in tumors based on a new radiofrequency
    procedure. J. Cancer Res. Clin. Oncol. 49: 590, 1979.
29. von Ardenne, M., Kell, E., Berechnung des dynamischen Aufheiz-
    prozesses in mehrschichtigen Modellgeweben bei Lokal-
    hyperthermie nach dem CMT-Selektotherm-Verfahren. Arch
    Geschwulstforsch, 49: 590, 1979.

RESULTS OF A PHASE I/II CLINICAL TRIAL OF FRACTIONATED HYPERTHERMIA

IN COMBINATION WITH LOW DOSE IONIZING RADIATION

Haim I. Bicher, M. D., Ph.D., Fred W. Hetzel, Ph.D.,
and Taljit S. Sandhu, Ph.D.

Department of Therapeutic Radiology, Henry Ford Hospital,
Detroit, Michigan 48202

FRACTIONATED HYPERTHEMIA

Abstract

This paper addresses, in part, the current status of hyperthermia as a new clincal modality and reports the results of a
large, prospective clinical trial employing microwave hyperthermia
in combination with low doses of ionizing radiation. In the
protocol employed, each treated area received 8 hyperthermia treatments of 1.5 hour combined with 1600 rad over a total period of 5
weeks. Patients were heated with microwaves of 915 or 300 MHz
employing external applicators or internal intracavitary antennas.
The results of this fractionation scheme are encouraging since in
121 fields that were treated completely according to protocol and
were available for follow-up for at least 2 months, complete
responses were observed in 65% of all cases, partial response in
30% and no response in only 5%. It is also important to note that
toxicity was minimal throughout the study.

Introduction

The use of hyperthermia as a clinical modality has taken great
strides in the past few years as more investigators realized the
importance of complete temperature and treatment documentation.

Recent studies (1-7) involving a combination of hyperthermia
and x-irradiation have made a serious effort to measure and docu-
ment the hyperthermia treatments more accurately. In most cases
a comparison with radiation alone controls is made. Kim et al.
(5) have treated 50 patients with a variety of cutaneous tumors.

Improved results are reported for both the radiosensitive (i.e.
mycosis fungoides) and radioresistant (i.e. melanoma) tumors with
the combined hyperthermia and radiation treatment as compared to
either of these modalities used alone. These authors report complete
disappearance of multiple recurrent melanoma nodules without unusual
normal skin reactions. However, combination therapy did produce
enhanced skin reactions in patients whose treated areas included
either a skin graft or heavily scarred skin from extensive surgery.

Hornback et al. (3) treated 72 patients with advanced cancer
using the combined therapy. Of the patients treated with hyperthermia prior to radiation therapy, 53% experienced complete remission of symptoms while in the group of patients treated with
heat following radiotherapy, 92% showed complete remission. Again
there was no set protocol and the radiation doses varied from 500
to 600 rad per day with total doses from 3000 to 6500 rads. Heat
treatments were given using 433.92 MHz microwaves. Although the
authors mention having attempted to measure tumor temperature during
these treatments, there is no mention of tumor temperatures achieved
in the patients.

Manning et al. (6) reported a very limited study combining
localized heat and radiation. The response rate for heat-radiation
combination was 80-90% compared with 50% response rate for heat
alone and radiation alone groups. The authors suggest a beneficial
therapeutic ratio and minimal side effects from the combined treatments.

Another limited study (7) treated two groups of patients with
radiotherapy alone, hyperthermia alone, and combined treatment.
One group of patients received 200-600 rad fractions, 2-5 times
per week to a total of 1800-2400 rad in 5-14 fractions. The
other group of patients received the combined thermoradiotherapy
treatments only, radiation fractions of 200-600 rad, 2-5 times a
week to a total of 2000-4800 rad in 6-20 fractions. Hyperthermic
treatments for both groups was 42-44°C, 2-3 times per week to a
maximum of ten sessions in four weeks. Hyperthermia treatments
were given using either 2450 or 915 MHz microwaves. The first
group of 8 patients, six patients experienced complete regression
of lesions treated with radiation plus hyperthermia within one
month of therapy. None of the tumors treated with hyperthermia
alone regressed completely. In the second group of patients 73%
showed tumor regression. Melanoma regressed completely in 2/4
cases. No adverse side effects were observed on normal tissue
from the combined treatment.

Another interesting study was reported by Arcangeli et al.
(1). In fifteen patients with multiple neck node metastases from
head and neck treated with either radiation alone or in combination
with hyperthermia. A total of 33 neck nodes were treated, 12 with

radiation alone and the rest with the combination.

The radiation schedule resulted in 46% complete response which
was enhanced to 85% complete response when combined with hyperthermia,
the remaining 15% showed partial response. It should be noted that
in the treatment schedule, when radiation was combined with hyperthermia, heat was applied immediately after the second daily fraction.
The authors did not observe any abnormal reactions in areas that
were treated with combined therapy.

In a preliminary publication (2) we reported an effective
fractionation regime using $45^{\circ}C$ regional hyperthermia combined with
low dose (1600 rads) x-irradiation, yielding an overall total
response rate of 65%. These results are now expanded to include an
enlarged series as well as introducing an intracavitary device for
the treatment of deep seated tumors.

The above mentioned clinical studies are both interesting and
encouraging. In addition, recent physiological evidence shows a
differential "breaking point" in blood flow in tumors as compared
to normal tissues which results in dramatic shifts in intratumor
pH (8). These observations may, in part, explain the results of
the clinical trial we are reporting here.

Method

The exact protocol followed has been reported in detail else-
where (2) (also RTOG protocol #78-06A). Briefly, treatment consisted of 4 fractions of hyperthermia alone followed after a one
week rest by 4 additional fractions of hyperthermia this time immediately following radiation. All treatments were separated by
72 hours following a Monday-Thursday or Tuesday-Friday pattern.
Each hyperthermia treatment was for $1\frac{1}{2}$ hours at the prescribed
temperature ($45^{\circ}C$ alone; $42^{\circ}C$ with radiation) and each radiation
dose was 400 rad. Therefore, treatment consisted of a total of
8 hyperthermia treatments and 1600 rad over a total period of 5
weeks.

Complete thermometry was performed during every patient
treatment employing microthermocouples (100μ). The microthermocouples were implanted in the tumor (whenever possible) and in
surrounding or overlying normal tissues. Throughout treatment,
temperature readings were taken at 5 minute intervals under "power-
off" conditions to eliminate any possible interference artifacts.

Heating was accomplished using either 915 or 300 MHz microwaves
delivered with partially dielectric loaded external beam applicators
or intracavitary antennas. In all cases air cooling was applied
either to the skin (external applicators) or to the jacket of the
antenna to minimize normal tissue heating (and hence damage). With

the variety of heating equipment available we have been able to
heat uniformly externally up to 7 cm in depth as well as internally
heating the head and neck, mediastinum and pelvis (1).

Results

At this time 178 patients have been treated at our clinic with
a multimodality regime involving hyperthermia administered in multifraction fashion (8 hyperthermia treatments per field). Since
many of these patients had multiple tumors, at least 250 tumors
have been treated (over 2,000 treatment sessions). Not all of them
fitted all criteria for inclusion in the specific protocol, but
among evaluable results the follwing can be cited:
    121 fields (tumors) were treated according to our 8
    fraction protocol with 1600 rads in 4 fractions. The
    final results show almost no toxicity, and a rate of
    65% of total responses and 30% partial response.
Further analysis of this series is shown in Tables I-VII.

Table I shows a summary of all the patients treated which
completed the entire protocol and were followed up at least two
months. Table II provides a breakdown of the summarized data by
histology. From this table it is clear that every histological
type treated does respond to this therapy.

Table III reports the results of our toxicity study employing
the intracavitary microwave antenna system. Following 212 (All
equipment was supplied by Medtra Inc., 1350 W. Bethune, Detroit,
Michigan, 48202.) treatment sessions of 1½ hours each, the only
observed toxicity was one central pneumonitis. Since response is
only evaluated after 2 months at this time only 14 patients are
evaluable (Table IV). Even in these patients with deep seated
tumors (mediastinum, pelvis) only 14% failed to respond.

Tables V-VII evaluate response to the combined modality in
different anatomical locations. In head and neck recurrences,
breast and chest wall, and skin tumors only a small percentage
(9%, 10% and 3% respectively) failed to respond to combined hyperthermia and radiation while total responses varied from 46% to 76%
yielding our reported average of 65.5% (Table I).

Discussion

As seen in the detailed response breakdown shown in Table II,
the hyperthermia-radiation fractionation regime chosen seems to
be at least partially successful in a wide variety of tumors. Detailed examination of the data shows essentially no treatment
toxicity with the antenna applicators (Table III) since 212 sessions
(318 hours) of treatment resulted in only one case of minimal
toxicity. During these treatments (Table IV) tumor response was

TABLE I   SUMMARY OF RESULTS

121 Fields Treated: (82 patients)

   Total Response   79 (65.5%)

   Partial Response   36 (29.7%)

   No Response   6 (5.0%)

Recurrence: Local: 5

                            Marginal: 3

Complications: Skin burns: 2 (completely healed)

                            Tongue & Pharynx
                                burns: 2 (completely healed)

                            Grand seizure: 1 (neck treatment)
                                         (epileptic patient)

TABLE II   RESULTS BY HISTOLOGY

HISTOLOGY	NO. OF FIELDS	RESPONSE	FOLLOW-UP (MONTHS)
Malignant Melanoma	19	9 Total	2 - 14
		7 Partial	
		3 No Response	
Malignant Lymphoma	8	8 Total	2 - 9
Squamous Cell Carcinoma	25	9 Total	2 - 8
		15 Partial	
		1 No Response	
Adenocarcinoma	60	48 Total	2 - 9
		10 Partial	
		2 No Response	
Other (Transitional Cell, Basal Cell, Glioma, Sarcoma)	9	5 Total	2 - 11
SUMMARY	121	79 Total	2 - 14
		36 Partial	
		6 No Response	

Total Response: No tumor at 2 months follow-up and thereafter

Partial Response: Tumor decreased in size to half or less at 2 months follow-up

TABLE III   RESULTS-INTRACAVITARY ANTENNA-TOXICITY

10	Complete	(Less Than)	2	Month	Follow	Up	10	ΔT	Each	100
14	Complete	(At Least)	2	Month	Follow	Up	8	ΔT	Each	112

TOTAL 212 Sessions

Toxicity - 1 Central Pneumonitis

ΔT = Hyperthermia Treatment of 1½ hours

TABLE IV   RESULTS-INTRACAVITARY ANTENNA-RESPONSE

14 PATIENTS - COMPLETE - ALIVE   AT   2   MONTHS

8 H y p e r t h e r m i a   T r e a t m e n t s

1600 Rads - 2 Weeks - 4 Fractions

TR 6   1 Local Recurrence

PR 6

NR 2

TABLE V   RESULTS–HEAD AND NECK PATIENTS

NECK RECURRENCES

Total Patients	Total Response	Partial Response	No Response	Recurrence
22	10	10	2	1

TABLE VI   BREAST AND CHEST WALL

Total No. of Fields	Total Response	Partial Response	No Response	No. of Incompletes
29	19	7	3	3

TABLE VII   SKIN TUMORS

Total No. of Fields	Total Response	Partial Response	No Response
33	25	7	1

seen in all but 2 cases. Site specific analysis (Tables V-VII)
also shows the relative effectiveness of this therapy regardless
of anatomical location.

The fractionation regime employed in this study (regional hyperthermia plus low dose radiation) should be compared with those
employed in other reported clinical trials.

In their study, Kim et al, (5) report 78% overall tumor control
rate after combined therapy as compared with 26% after radiation
alone. These investigators utilized two heating methods. Some
patients with tumors on extremities were heated by immersion in
waterbath. The rest of the patients were treated using RF (27.12
MHz) inductive heating. It should be pointed out that there is a
great deal of variation in both the radiation dose and the hyperthermia treatment duration as well as in the number of fractions.
The radiation dose employed varied from 800 rad in two fractions
for melanoma to 2400 rad in 8 fractions for Kaposi's sarcoma.
Similarly hyperthermia (43.5°C) treatments varied from 2 fractions
of 30 minutes for melanoma to 5 fractions of 60 minutes for mycosis
fungoides. The hyperthermia treatments followed immediately the
radiation treatments in all cases. This data does not suggest any
particular treatment schedule for a particular tumor. The study
does, however, demonstrate the improved effectiveness of combined
thermoradiotheapy as compared to hyperthermia or radiation alone.

In the study by Manning et al. (6), of the 40 patients treated
with hyperthermia, four were treated in combination with radiation.
Each had a minimum of 3 nodules. One nodule received a heat treatment of 43°C for 40 minutes using radiofrequency currents. Another
nodule received radiation alone from two radium needles to a dose
of 4000 rads in 100 hours. A third lesion had the same dose plus
simultaneous heat to 43°C for 40 minutes using radium needles as
heating electrodes. A 30-40% increase in response was observed
for the combination therapy.

Arcangeli and co-workers (1) employed a rather unique technique
in their protocol. Hyperthermia was induced by 500 MHz microwaves
using a non contact applicator. These investigators used a very
interesting fractional scheme. Described as a multiple daily
fractional (MDF) scheme, it consisted of 200 + 150 + 150 rad/day,
4-5 hours interval between fractions, 5 days per week, up to a
total of 4000/7000 rad. All the lesions were irradiated with the
same total dose, whether or not they received hyperthermia. Again
a 40% increase in response was seen for the combined modality
therapy.

Johnson et al. (4) conducted a pilot study to evaluate normal
skin and melanoma tumor thermal enhancement ratios of 41.5 to 42°C
hyperthermia with radiation. The response of normal skin to the

treatment was measured by evaluating the degree of erythema according to a numerical scoring system. Tumor response was assessed by measuring tumor diameter. Although the study was not conclusive about the thermal enhancement ratio, it did bring to light some of the problems associated with obtaining useful clinical data. The study involved patients with multiple metastatic melanoma lesions. At least three lesions were chosen on each patient. The patients were divided into three groups and given one, 3 or 4 fractions, with a minimum of 72 hours interval between each fraction. Radiation dose per fraction for different lesions on a patient varied from 500 to 900 rad. In some cases single fractions of 1000, 1200 or 1300 rad were used. On all patients one lesion was heated immediately following radiation therapy and the other two or more lesions treated with radiation alone were used for comparison. Hyperthermia treatments were administered using 915 MHz direct contact microwave applicators (4). Duration of hyperthermia treatments varied between 1 and 2 hours at 41.5 - 42.0°C.

Skin enhancement ratio (SER) and thermal enhancement ratio (TER) could be evaluated only for a limited number of patients because of lack of follow up data. SER values varied for 1.2 to 1.7 while TER values in most cases were 1.3. This study demonstrated, however, that superficial tumors up to 4 cm in diameter and 2 cm in depth could be treated with an accuracy of $\pm$ 0.5°C either during, or after radiation with 915 MHz microwaves.

The study reported here as well as the results of other investigators tend to indicate the relative effectiveness and lack of overall adverse effects from combined hyperthermia and radiation. Further prospective, site specific trials are now planned or in progress to further evaluate both the safety and effectiveness of fractionated hyperthermia and radiation. In addition, the patients already treated will continue to be followed at 2 month intervals.

REFERENCES

1. Arcangeli, G., Barni, E., Dividalli, A., et al. Effectiveness of microwave hyperthermia combined with ionizing radiation: clinical results on neck node metastases. Int. J. Radiat. Oncol. Biol. Phys. 1980; 6: 143-148.
2. Bicher, H. I., Sandhu, T. S., Hetzel, F. W. Hyperthermia and radiation in combination: a clinical fractionation regime. Int. J. Radiat. Oncol. Biol. Phys. 1980; 6: 867-870.
3. Hornback, N. B., Shupe, R. E., Homayon, S., et al. Preliminary clinical results of combined 433 MHz microwave therapy and radiation therapy on patients with advanced cancer. Cancer 1977; 40: 2354-2863.
4. Johnson, R. J. R., Sandhu, T. S., Hetzel, F. W., et al. A pilot study to investigate the therapeutic ratio of 41.5-42.0 C hyperthermia radiation. Int. J. Radiat. Oncol.

Biol. Phys. 1979; 5: 947-953.
5. Kim, J. H., Hahn, E. W., Benjamin, F. J.   Treatment of super-
     ficial cancers by combination hyperthermia and radiation
     therapy.   Clin. Bul. 1979; 9: 13-16.
6. Manning, M. R., Cetas, T., Boone, M. L. M., Miller, R. C.
     Clinical hyperthermia: results of the phase I clinical
     trial combining localized hyperthermia with or without
     radiation.   (Abstr.) Int. J. Radiat. Oncol. Biol. Phys.
     1979; 5: S2: 173.
7. U. R., Noell, K. T., Woodward, K. T. et al.   Microwave-induced
     local hyperthermia in combination with radiotherapy of
     human malignant tumors.   Cancer 1980; 45: 638-646.
8. Bicher, H. I., Hetzel, F. W., Sandhu, T. S., et al.   Effects
     of hyperthermia on normal and tumor microenvironment.
     Radiology 1980; 137: 523-530.

ADJUVANT HYPERTHERMIA IN THE IRRADIATION OF METASTATIC TUMOR MASSES

UTILIZING 2450 MHz MICROWAVES

John T. Fazekas, M. D., Rudolph E. Nerlinger, B. S.,
Frank M. Waterman, Ph.D., Dennis B. Leeper, Ph.D.

Department of Radiation Therapy and Nuclear Medicine
Thomas Jefferson University Hospital
Philadelphia, Pennsylvania 19107

INTRODUCTION

Clinical interest in hyperthermia as a safe and effective adjuvant to irradiation in cancer therapy continues to heighten. The review of experimental and clinical studies by Overgaard suggests that the optimal thermal enhancement ratio (TER) may be obtained by simultaneous administration of both modalities; however, an improvement in therapeutic ratio (tumor effect vs. skin effect) may be best attained by sequential administration of radiotherapy and hyperthermia and with sessions separated by intervals of three hours or longer. Most clinical studies have either administered the heat shortly before irradiation therapy (Kim et al., Marmor and Hahn, Manning et al.) or immediately after (Bicher et al., Perez et al., Arcangeli et al., and Luk).

Overgaard, and Stewart and Denecamp have shown that heat administration prior to irradiation (heat plus XRT) tends to enhance the damage to skin compared to the opposite sequence (XRT plus heat). If one evaluates reported tumor responses, irrespective of normal tissue damage, utilizing combined hyperthermia-irradiation in treating superficial tumor deposits, results among all investigators are similar. Treating in the temperature range of 42.5-44.0°C in combination with modest doses of irradiation (generally 3000 + 1000 rad), a combined tumor response (complete and partial) in the 50-80% range is reported (2, 3, 4, 5, 6, 7, 8); however, minimal clinical information is available on skin effect within these various programs. This report outlines the techniques and results obtained among 87 patients entered in a phase II pilot program combined radiation therapy and immediate 42.5-43.5°C heating for

99

40-50 minutes in superficially recurrent tumor masses treated with palliative intent.

METHODS AND MATERIALS

The clinical criteria for consideration of entry into this phase II pilot included the following seven conditions:
1.   Skin, subcutaneous, or nodal tumor deposit(s) present with or without other manifestations of cancer. Histologic proof of malignancy is requred; however, the tumor nodule under consideration for hyperthermia may not necessarily be biopsied.
2.   Thickness of individual tumor deposit(s) generally less than 3 cm. as determined by caliper measurements or radiographic (including C. T. and ultrasound) studies.
3.   Tumor deposits representing either recurrent or metastatic cancer, having failed prior treatment modalities (surgery, chemotherapy and/or irradiation).
4.   Administration of heat must be technically feasible based upon anatomic area, extent of tumor in relationship to applicator size (10 cm. x 15 cm.) and location of major cooling vessels.
5.   Patients must sign informed consent allowing probe placement and agreeing to the experimental modality.
6.   Patients must have a Karnofsky score of 50 or beyond and have life expectancy of at least three months.
7.   Concomitant chemotherapy or hormonal manipulations are allowed if the systemic regimen is not altered for one month prior to consideration of hyperthermia.

Between January 1980 and December 1981, 87 patients were accepted into the program according to the above criteria. Sites and histologies of the cases entered into this study are shown in Table 1. The majority of the 87 patients (57) bore carcinomas (adeno or squamous), with 21 melanoma deposits representing the second highest category. Chest wall deposits were the predominant anatomic site, accounting for 32 of the 87 patients treated in this pilot.

Each patient received two or three fractions per week of radiotherapy to the gross disease with 1-2 cm. margins utilizing appropriate electron beam energies that encompassed the deepest portion of measurable tumor within the 80% isodose. Individual fractions of 225-275 rad were given for squamous and adenocarcinomas, and 350-400 rad for melanomas, to total doses of 2500-4000 rad. Obviously, pre-existing therapies (e.g. prior radiotherapy to region under treatment or concomitant chemotherapy) largely mandate the dosage of radiotherapy administered. The average tumor dose amongst these 87 patients was a modest 2700 rad in 20 elapsed days. Hyperthermia (as defined by intralesional tumor temperatures) was administered twice weekly for 40-50 minute sessions, maintaining the tumor temperature in the 42.5-44.5°C whenever possible for a minimum of 35 minutes per session. Achievement of effective hyper-

TABLE 1

SITES TREATED

Chest wall deposits		32
Recurrent breast	(28)	
Other, including melanoma	(4)	
Neck/supraclavicular deposts (skin or nodes)		31
Miscellaneous sites		24
	Total	87

HISTOLOGIES

Carcinomas (adeno/squamous)		57
Melanoma		21
Lymphoma		3
Sarcoma		6
	Total	87

thermia conditions (42.5°C or beyond) generally requires 5-10 minutes
at an applied power of 30-50 watts, depending upon blood flow, tumor
size, and other physiologic factors. A total of 6-8 heating sessions
are administered over a 3-3½ week period.

Our current approach utilizes direct contact microwave applicators operated at 2450 MHz with a maximum power of 100 watts.
Thermostatically controlled circulating water is used for surface
cooling. The water temperature is typically maintained at 44°C
for tumors with no overlying normal tissue. When tumor deposits
are subcutaneous or below, colder water temperatures are utilized
to spare the skin while allowing the power output to be increased.
In the latter case, our aim is to keep the skin temperature below
the therapeutic range while heating the deeper tumor tissue. The
surface water bag also aids in coupling the microwave power to the
tissue.

Sterile I.V. catheters (16-18 g, Becton-Dickinson) are placed
within the tumor mass under local anesthesia (Lidocaine without
epinephrine) at the beginning of each hyperthermia session for
insertion of thermometer probes. Whenever feasible, the probe(s)
are placed near the tumor center at depths ranging from 0.5 to 2.5
cm. below the skin. Surface temperatures are also monitored.

During the early phase of this program, only thermocouples
were available for temperature measurements. Since accurate
measurements could be obtained only with the power off, tumor
temperatures were recorded every five minutes. In early 1981,
we acquired a Luxtron Model 100D fluoroptic thermometer which is
electrically non-conductive and non-perturbing in radiofrequency or
microwave fields. Later in 1981, we acquired a minimally perturbing
Vitek probe. This probe consists of two pairs of very high resistance plastic leads having a conductivity only slightly greater
than tissue.

Stability has been a problem with the Luxtron probe; however,
the drift is reduced to about 0.1°C per hour after a 4-hour warm-
up period. Another problem is that the instrument is accurate
only at the temperature at which it is calibrated. Temperatures
five degrees higher or lower may be in error by a few tenths of a
degree. The Vitek, on the other hand, has proven to be accurate to
better than 0.1°C per month. The only disadvantage of the Vitek
probe is that its larger diameter requires a 16 gauge needle for
insertion of the probe.

The Vitek and thermocouple probes are periodically calibrated
by use of a mercury thermometer having a calibration traceable to
the National Bureau of Standards and circulating water bath that
maintains the water temperature to within 0.03°C. Prior to, and
immediately after, each patient treatment the calibrations of Vitek,

Luxtron and thermocouple probes are checked in the water bath.

During patient treatments, the temperatures of the Vitek and
Luxtron probes are continuously recorded on a strip chart recorder.
In addition, the thermal washout, or the decrease of temperature
with time, is presently recorded at the conclusion of each patient
treatment. This data provides an indication of the blood flow rate
in the tumor since the rate of temperature decrease is proportional
to the product of the blood flow rate and the difference between
the temperatures of the tissue and incoming blood. Thermal washout
measurements of 1-2 minutes duration are also made during selective
treatment sessions to study the change in blood flow rate with time
and temperature.

RESULTS

Tumor regression was the main criteria investigated by this
hyperthermia pilot. Due to the advanced, usually metastatic
nature of the patient population, longterm survival was neither
expected nor generally observed. A second and equally important
parameter was the effect (damage) of normal skin resultant form the
combined effects of hyperthermia and irradiation. Whenever feasible,
autologous controls (x-ray therapy only) were included to identical
tumor doses in similar cancer deposits located within another anatomic
region. Since these control deposits were available in only nine
cases, no generalization can be made regarding response/therapeutic
gain parameters.

Twenty-four patients were inevaluable either due to early
death (4), failure to consistently attain adequate temperature (6),
failure to complete the program (8), or were lost to follow-up (6).
Tumor response was determined by caliper measurements (l x w).
Absence of all visible and palpable tumor was evaluated as a complete
response (CR); 50% or greater tumor regression as a partial response
(PR). Response according to histologic subtype (Table 2) reveals
the highest CR and combined response (CR + PR) for melanoma deposits
(53% and 73% respectively), although the total number of cases is
small (21 entered, 15 evaluable). To what degree individual
fractionation has added to response is unclear; however, the recent
review of Katz would suggest that the total doses and the dose-
fractionation schemas utilized in our pilot (3600-4000 rad at 350-
400 rad fraction) results in clearance rates in the 0-29% range, well
below the 53% CR observed in our pilot series.

Carcinomas (superficial deposits of recurrent/metastatic adeno
or squamous types) were below melanomas in response (58% CR + PR,
27% CR) similar to the published results of Luk and Perez et al.
for similar lesions and anatomic sites. Our limited experience with
sarcomas has been uniformly poor.

TABLE 2

RESPONSE BY HISTOLOGIC SUBTYPE

Carcinomas	No.
No response	20
Partial response	15
Complete response	13
Not evaluable	9
Total cases	57
Total evaluable pts	48

Melanomas	No.
No response	4
Partial response	3
Complete response	8
Not evaluable	6
Total cases	21
Total evaluable pts	15

Tumor response was also analyzed by anatomic region. Skin overlying chest wall appears to be the most favorable and suitable for 2450 MHz microwave hyperthermia. Seventy percent of all CR's and 60% of the PR's occurred within the chest wall while only 9 of the 20 NR's (<50% shrinkage) bore tumor masses upon or within this structure. Since our initial clinical observations (13) documented effective heating (42°C or greater) to a depth of 2 cm. with 2450 MHz microwaves, our clinical observations are probably due to the fact that the chest wall is thin and accessible.

Blood flow rates obtained from thermal washout measurements in relatively small superficial tumors indicate that the blood flow rate increases by about a factor of three during the initial temperature rise to the therapeutic region. Thereafter, the flow rate remains relatively constant. The absolute values of the blood flow rates obtained vary from about 30 to 100 ml/100 gm min. Since the model used to calculate the flow rate contains several assumptions, we are constructing a dynamic phantom to test the re-liability of the model.

DISCUSSION

In addition to the clinically important observations regarding tumor response utilizing microwave (2450 MHz) hyperthermia adjuvant to modest doses of radiotherapy, response rate variations by anatomic site and histologic type raise provocative questions. Are melanoma deposits a priori more heat sensitive than are other cancerous subtypes like squamous/adeno carcinomas? Are tumor deposits upon the chest wall region more amenable to therapy or is tumor in that anatomic region apparently more prone to thermal damage for biological reasons? Why have hyperthermia efforts been uniformly futile in sarcomatous deposits?

While answers to these questions are yet unavailable, this pilot has instructed us in these areas:
1) 2450 MHz microwave hyperthermia is quite effective for tumor deposits of melanoma and carcinoma but tumor thickness can be no more than 2.5 cm.
2) Skin cooling by circulating water prevents serious skin complications and aids in improving the therapeutic ratio.
3) Previous therapies, including prior radiotherapy, does not prevent the application of effective therapy (irradiation followed by heat) since no serious late skin effects (necrosis, telangectasias, fibrosis) were observed during the limited follow-up of these 87 patients (1-20 mo.).
4) Utilizing non-perturbing intralesional thermal probes (Vitek or Luxtron), important information on thermal washout can be obtained allowing translation of this data into estimates of tumor blood flow (14). Alterations of these haematodynamic parameters during treatment may yield valuable clues to the vascular effects of clinical hyperthermia.

REFERENCES

1. Overgaard, J. Fractionated radiation and hyperthermia.
   Experimental and clinical studies. Cancer 48:1116-1123,
   1981.
2. Kim, J. H., Hahn, E. W., Tokita, N. Combination hyperthermia
   and radiation therapy for cutaneous malignant melanoma.
   Cancer 41:2143-2148, 1978.
3. Marmor, J. B., Hahn, G. M. Combined radiation and hyperthermia
   in superficial human tumors. Cancer 47: 1986-1991, 1980.
4. Manning, M. R., Cetas, T. C., Miller, R. C., Oleson, J. R.,
   Connor, W. G., Gerner, E. W. Clinical hypertheramia:
   Results of a Phase I trial employing hyperthermia alone
   or in combination with external beam or interstitial
   radiotherapy. Cancer 49:205-216, 1982.
5. Bicher, H. I., Sandhu, T. S., Hetzel, F. W. Hyperthermia and
   radiation in combination: A clinical fractionation regimen.
   Int. J. Radiat. Oncol. Biol. Phys. 6:867-870, 1980.
6. Perez, C. A., Kopecky, W., Baglan, R., Rao, D. V., Johnson,
   R. Local microwave hyperthermia in cancer therapy.
   Preliminary report. Henry Ford Hospital Med. J. 29:16-23,
   1981.
7. Arcangeli, G., Barni, E., Cividallo, A., Mauro, F., Morelli,
   D., Nervi, C., Spano, M., Tabocchini, A. Effectiveness
   of microwave hyperthermia combined with inionizing radiation: Clinical results on neck node metastases. Int. J.
   Radiat. Oncol. Biol. Phys. 6:143-148, 1980.
8. Luk, K. H. An updated analysis of microwave hyperthermia at
   2450 Megahertz and 915 Megahertz frequencies. Henry Ford
   Hospital Med. J. 29:28-31, 1981.
9. Overgaard, J. Simultaneous and sequential hyperthermia and
   radiation treatment of an experimental tumor and its
   surrounding normal tissue in vivo. Int. J. Radiat. Oncol.
   Biol. Phys. 6:1507-1517, 1980.
10. Stewart, F. A., Denekamp, J. Sensitization of mouse skin to
    X irradiation by moderate heating. Radiology 123:195-200,
    1977.
11. Henle, K. J., Leeper, D. B. Interaction of hyperthermia and
    radiation in CHO cells: Recovery kinetics. Radiat. Res.
    66:505-518, 1976.
12. Katz, H. R. The results of different fractionation schemes in
    the palliative irradiation of metastatic melanoma. Int.
    J. Radiat. Oncol. Biol. Phys. 7:907-911, 1981.
13. Fazekas, J. T., Nerlinger, R. E. Localized hyperthermia
    adjuvant to irradiation in superficial recurrent car-
    cinomas: A preliminary report on 46 patients. Int. J.
    Radiat. Oncol. Biol. Phys. 7:1457-1463, 1981.

14. Waterman, F. M., Fazekas, J., Nerlinger, R. E., Leeper, D. B.
    Blood flow rates in human tumors during hyperthermia
    treatments as indicated by thermal washout. To be
    presented at the 2nd Ann. Meeting of the N. Am. Hyper-
    thermia Group (NAHG), Salt Lake City, Utah, April, 1982.

FURTHER STUDIES ON THE NATURE OF THE BIPHASIC RADIATION SURVIVAL

RESPONSE OF CHINESE HAMSTER CELLS V-79-753B TO MOLECULAR OXYGEN

Barbara C. Millar, E. Martin Fielden and Sally Jinks

Radiobiology Unit, Division of Physics. Institute of
Cancer Research
Clifton Avenue, Sutton, Surrey, UK

INTRODUCTION

We have previously reported that for Chinese hamster cells,
V-79-753B, irradiated as monolayer cultures at room temperature
in phosphate buffered saline (PBSA), the radiation survival response
is biphasic with respect to oxygen concentration (1). At oxygen
concentrations between 1.5 and 7.0 µM sensitization is constant,
equivalent to an oxygen enhancement ratio of 1.9 compared with the
full oxygen enhancement ratio of 3.1. This region of constant
sensitization has been designated the "plateau". Additionally,
examination of the initial yield of single strand breaks (ssb) in
the irradiated DNA of this cell line showed that the full oxygen
effect was produced at an oxygen concentration of 1.5 µM, the start
of the "plateau" in terms of cell survival (2). Whilst a similar
biphasic survival response has been seen for bacterial spores
irradiated in the presence of different concentrations of oxygen
(3), there is as yet no other example for either bacterial (4) or
mammalian cells (5,6). The equation developed by Howard-Flanders
and Alpher (7), which postulates that oxygen is in simple competition
with target repair reactions, cannot be applied to this cell line.
Furthermore, the shape of the survival response curve is not unique
to molecular oxygen. When hypoxic cells are irradiated in the
presence of different concentrations of radiosensitizers the
radiation survival response is also biphasic as a function of the
concentration of sensitizer (2). Additionally, using a rapid-mix
technique sensitization by misonidazole has been shown to occur by
two time resolvable components (8).

The present report is concerned with attempts to investigate
factors that may influence the biphasic nature of the radiation

survival curve of Chinese hamster V-79-753B cells. We have considered the effect of temperature, growth media, sulphydryl levels and respiratory effects to determine whether the "plateau" can be modified or its presence accounted for.

MATERIALS AND METHODS

The routine handling of cells and experimental design have been described previously (9, 1, 2). All experiments were done on 61 mM glass Petri dishes in full growth medium supplemented with 15% foetal bovine serum and 20 mM Hepes buffer unless indicated in the text. Data were taken from full survival curves and all experiments were carried out at least twice. Where there was evidence of similar amounts of sensitization for different concentrations of oxygen or misonidazole, additional experiments were done to compare these concentrations on a "same day" basis. Each day's experiment consisted of a control curve for hypoxic cells and curves using increasing concentrations of oxygen or misonidazole where appropriate. The hypoxic survival curve was always carried out first, followed by increasing concentrations of oxygen, to reduce the possibility that the gas line would become contaminated with trace amounts of oxygen.

Cells were plated out in the morning and experiments commenced approximately 5.5 hours later, this interval being set by the availability of the radiation source. This time interval did not affect the multiplicity of the plated cells, i.e. no division had occurred. Irradiations were carried out using a Cobalt-60 source. The dose rate was ~3.7 Gray min^{-1} for cultures irradiated at room temperature and ~5.0 Gray min^{-1} for cultures irradiated at 37°C. This difference is dictated by the geometry of the 37°C irradiation jig. All irradiations were done in sealed "Dural" containers containing 3 Petri dishes/irradiation sample. Cultures were degassed for 15 minutes prior to irradiation. The volume of liquid on each dish was 0.5 ml and gases were pre-humidified by bubbling through distilled water to prevent the cultures from drying. Samples to be irradiated at 37°C were held on a temperature-controlled plate throughout the gassing period. After irradiation the medium/PBSA was aspirated from the dishes and replaced with 2.0 ml fresh growth medium. When cells had been exposed to cyanide, the mono-layer was washed once with PBSA prior to addition of fresh growth medium. Cultures were incubated for 6-7 days to allow colony formation at which time the medium was removed, the colonies fixed the ethanol and stained with methylene blue.

Pooled data from repeat experiments were analysed by computer CDC400 using the multitarget equation to give errors on D_0 (10). Computer analysis to the multitarget equation was done to remove subjective bias and not as an indication of the underlying mechanism.

Chemicals. Gas mixtures prepared volumetrically and of

certified composition (O_2 concentration within 10% of stated) were
supplied by BOC (England). Each gas mixture was checked by a
"Thermox I" meter (Thermox Instruments Inc., Pittsburgh, Pa., USA).
The concentration of oxygen in aqueous solution was calculated using
solubility constants for oxygen at different temperatures (11).

Diamide was supplied from Sigma Chemical Co. Ltd. (Poole,
Dorset, England), potassium cyanide (AR) from Hopkins and Williams
(Chadwell Heath, Essex, England) and misonidazole was a gift from
Roche Products Ltd. (Welwyn Garden City, Herts, England).

RESULTS

A possible explanation for the constant radiation sensitization
seen for V-79-753B cells using oxygen concentrations between 1.5
and 7.0 μM at room temperature is that the sulphydryl level in the
cells may change as a function of time after plating. This has been
reported by Cullen et al. for Erlich Ascites cells (12). Since
experiments with V-79-753B cells follow a similar time course and
gas mixtures are used in succession from lowest oxygen concentration
to higher oxygen concentrations, this possibility was examined by
irradiating cells in full growth medium, 5.5, 6.5 and 7.5 hours
after plating, in 4.6 μM oxygen. This oxygen concentration was
chosen because variations in SH content would be expected to produce
the greatest effect on radiation sensitivity at the centre of the
"plateau" in the slope ratio SR versus oxygen concentration curve.
The data in Fig. 1 show the effect of irradiating cells at these
time intervals. There was no appreciable difference in the amount
of sensitization produced by 4.6 μM oxygen when cells were irradiated
5.5, 6.5 or 7.5 hr. after plating. Thus changes in SH level during
this period cannot explain the constant SR seen at O_2 concentrations
between 1.5 μM and 7.0 μM.

The data points in Fig. 2 are averaged from the pooled data of
all the experiments at given O_2 concentrations on the survival of
V-79-753B cells irradiated at 37°C in full growth medium. As the
concentration of oxygen was increased in the medium there was
progressively more sensitization but at oxygen concentrations of
2.0 μM and 3.0 μM the amount of sensitization was similar, equivalent
to an SR of approximately 1.9 (see Table 1). The curves in Fig. 2
are fitted by eye; however the data (from the same experiments)
in Table 1 have been subjected to computer analysis as described.
In both cases the coincidence of the data at 2 and 3 μM O_2 is
appropriate. Above 3.0 μM oxygen there was progressively more
sensitization until the maximum oxygen enhancement ratio was
reached at 11 μM oxygen. The data from Table 1 are plotted in
Fig. 3 as the slope ratio (SR) versus oxygen concentration together
with similar data from experiments carried out at room temperature
(20°C ± 1°C) in full growth medium. At the lower temperature the
shape of the slope ratio versus oxygen concentration curve is in

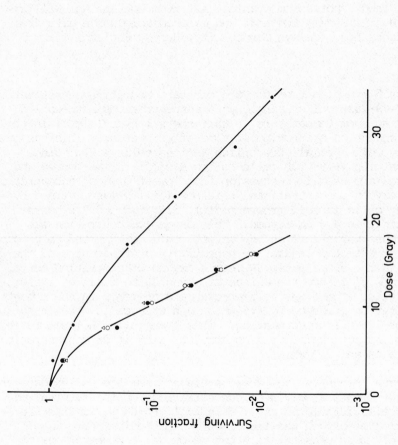

Fig. 1.   Effect of time after plating on the radiation survival of Chinese hamster cells V79-753B at room temperature in full growth medium. ○, cultures irradiated 5.5 hr. after plating; △, cultures irradiated 6.5 hr. after plating; ●, cultures irradiated 7.5 hr. after plating.

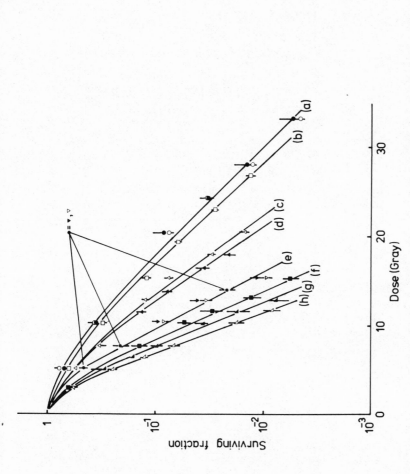

Fig. 2. Effect of O₂ on the radiation survival of Chinese hamster cells, V79-753B at 37°C in full growth medium. (a) ● N₂, ○ 0.095 μM O₂; (b) □, 0.61 μM O₂; (c) △, 0.81 μM O₂; (d) ▲, 1.16 μM O₂; (e) ▽, 2.0 μM O₂; (f) ▼, 3.0 μM O₂; ■, 4.725 μM O₂; (g) ▲, 8.14 μM O₂; (h) △, 11.92, 21.84, 54.39, 97.8 μM O₂ and air.

Table 1

Effect of O_2 on sensitization at 37°C in ME-15

(a) gas phase VPPM	Concentration of O_2 (b) in the medium (μM)	D_o (rad)	Slope ratio	$\dfrac{D_{o}(N_2)}{D_o}$
<6 (N_2 response)	0.0	527 ± 29	1.0	a
90	0.095	514 ± 14	1.03	b
580	0.61	480 ± 18	1.1	c
775	0.81	413 ± 30	1.28	d
1100	1.16	359 ± 21	1.47	
2300	2.0	276 ± 24	1.91	e
3200	3.05	285 ± 15	1.85	f
5500	4.725	230 ± 14	2.29	g
8800	8.14	218 ± 14	2.42	
1.23 x 10⁴	10.92	181 ± 7	2.92	
2.6 x 10⁴	21.84	178 ± 5	2.96	h
6 x 10⁴	54.39	186 ± 7	2.83	
9.31 x 10⁴	97.8	166 ± 6	3.18	
Air (2 x 10⁵)	252	178 ± 10	2.96	

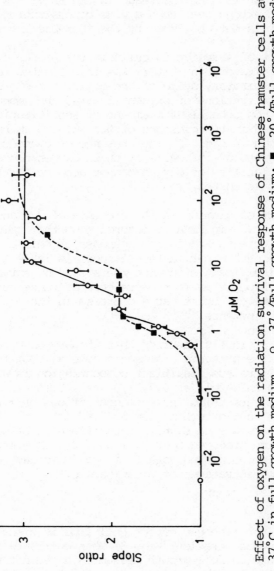

Fig. 3. Effect of oxygen on the radiation survival response of Chinese hamster cells at 37°C in full growth medium. ○, 37°/Full growth medium; ■, 20°/Full growth medium.

good agreement with previously published data (1) for the survival
of this cell line in PBSA. Thus the "plateau" cannot be ascribed
to an artifact due to irradiating cells in buffer rather than growth
medium. Also, whilst the "plateau" in the SR versus concentration
curve does not extend over such a wide concentration range at $37^{O}C$
as at $20^{O}C$, it is not abolished by the increase in temperature.

The effect of irradiating cells in the presence of potassium
cyanide (a respiratory inhibitor) was investigated to determine
whether the respiratory state of the cells in the presence of
different concentrations of oxygen affected the amount of oxygen
available and consequently the amount of sensitization. Data for
cells irradiated in the presence of 0.6 μM, 2.0 μM and 3.0 μM
oxygen are shown in Fig. 4. The presence of cyanide did not affect
the radiation response of cells at these oxygen concentrations.
Thus, the availability of oxygen cannot account for the shape of
survival response curves.

The effect of diamide in the presence of 2.0 and 3.0 μM oxygen
was examined at 37° in PBSA to determine whether removal of endogenous
sulphydryl affects the radiation response of cells. Computed data
from two "same day" experiments are shown in Table 2. Diamide
produced no significant effect on the slopes of survival curves
irradiated in hypoxia or in the presence of these concentrations
of oxygen. However, there was a decrease in the extrapolation
number in each instance.

We have previously reported that when hypoxic cells are
irradiated in the presence of misonidazole at room temperature the
shape of the SR versus sensitizer concentration is also biphasic
(2). Using misonidazole at 0.7, 1.0 and 2.0 mM the SR is ~1.9.
Similar experiments using these concentrations of misonidazole were
carried out in full growth medium at $37^{O}C$ (Fig. 5). At this higher
temperature there was no significant difference between the amount
of sensitization produced by 0.7, 1.0 or 2.0 mM misonidazole SR
~1.9. Fig. 5 shows pooled data from two "same day" experiments
using these concentrations of misonidazole.

DISCUSSION

The survival response of our cell line is biphasic as a function
of the oxygen concentration (Fig. 3) when cells are irradiated at
room temperature in full growth medium in agreement with earlier
results in PBSA (2), thus showing that the "plateau" cannot be
attributed to a medium defect at the time of irradiation.

Cullen et al. (12) reported that for in vitro cultured Erlich
ascites cells the non-protein sulphydryl levels (NPSH) rose by a
factor of three during the first two hours after plating into full
growth medium. This presumably reflects the difference in NPSH

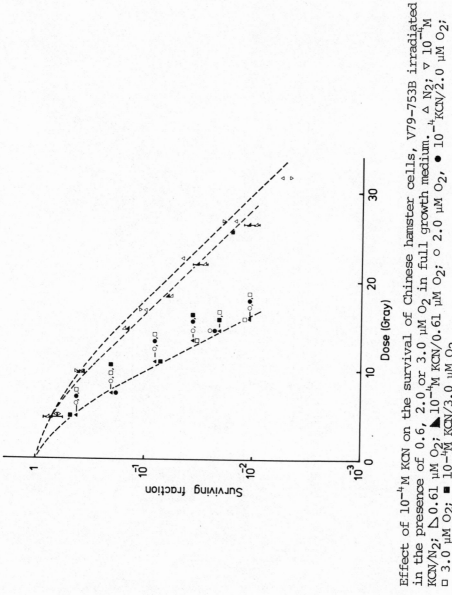

Fig. 4. Effect of 10^{-4} M KCN on the survival of Chinese hamster cells, V79-753B irradiated in the presence of 0.6, 2.0 or 3.0 μM O_2 in full growth medium. △ N_2; ▽ 10^{-4}M KCN/N_2; △ 0.61 μM O_2; ▲ 10^{-4}M KCN/0.61 μM O_2; ○ 2.0 μM O_2, ● 10^{-4} KCN/2.0 μM O_2; □ 3.0 μM O_2; ■ 10^{-4}M KCN/3.0 μM O_2

Table 2

Effect of Diamide on sensitization of V-79 cells in the
presence of 2.0 μM or 3.0 μM oxygen

	D_o(rad)	n	SR
N_2	522 ± 27	2.86 ± 0.7	1.00
N_2 + 25 μM Diamide	514 ± 15	1.09 ± 0.11	1.02
2 μM O_2	264 ± 30	4.08 ± 0.3	1.98
2 μM O_2 + 25 μM Diamide	269 ± 24	2.1 ± 0.8	1.91
3 μM O_2	273 ± 6	4.2 ± 0.5	1.91
3 μM O_2 + 25 μM Diamide	272 ± 16	2.08 ± 0.6	1.89

Effect principally on n;   no appreciable effect on D_o.

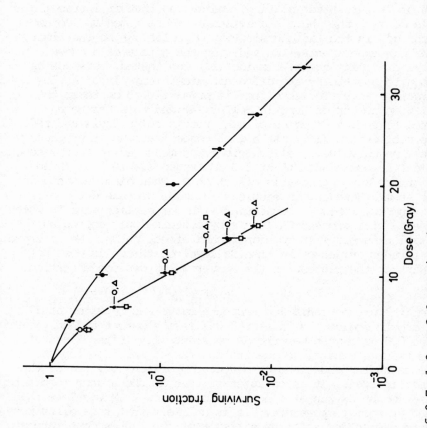

Fig. 5.   Effect of 0.7, 1.0 or 2.0 mM misonidazole on the radiation survival of Chinese hamster cells V79-753B at 37°C in full growth medium. ○, 0.7 mM misonidazole; △, 1.0 mM misonidazole; □, 2.0 mM misonidazole; ●, N₂ control.

levels between "old" cultures and exponential growth conditions.
Since at least exogenous SH levels affect the radiation response of
our cell line (13) it was necessary to check whether the effect
noted by Cullen et al. (12) was occurring in our system, particularly
since the experiments on any one day were done in ascending order
of oxygen concentration. Thus a fortuitous change in SH level over
a given range of oxygen concentration might have influenced the
results. However, the data in Fig. 1 show that there was no
significant difference between the survival of cells irradiated
5.5, 6.5 or 7.5 hr. after plating, indicating that if intracellular
SH levels do vary they have stabilized at these times and do not
effect changes in the radiosensitivity of cells during the time
course of our experiments. In addition the effect of a known
sulphydryl oxidizing agent, diamide (14) was tested. Diamide has
been shown to operate by two different mechanisms (15). At low
concentrations in vitro its effect is primarily to decrease the
extrapolation number of hypoxic cells (16) and this has been
attributed to the oxidization of non-protein sulphydryls and reduced
pyridine nucleotides (17). At higher concentrations it progressively
decreases the D_O value. Cell survival was measured in the presence
of diamide in anoxia and 2.0 or 3.0 µM oxygen (Table 2). In no
case was there any appreciable effect on D_O when diamide was added
to the system. However, in each case diamide decreased the extrapolation number. This is consistent with our earlier work in which
the presence of increased SH levels by cysteine only increased the
extrapolation number with no significant effect on D_O. We interpret
this as further evidence that the SH level of the cells does not
play a part in the plateau in the SR versus oxygen concentration
curve.

When the oxygen-radiation response curve was repeated at 37^OC
in full growth medium the "plateau" was less apparent and only over
the range 2.3 µM oxygen was the SR constant ~1.9 (Figs. 2 and 3).
Although this is a narrow concentration range, multiple repeat
experiments under conditions or direct comparison convince us that
the effect is real. It is of interest that at the higher temperature
sensitization by oxygen at concentrations below 2 µM was less than
that seen at room temperature. It is unlikely that this differnece
was due to oxygen depletion as a result of the higher dose rate at
37° is lower than at room temperature due to a higher rate of
metabolism. If this is the case such metabolism does not involve
respiration since there was no change in the survival response of
cells irradiated in the presence of 10^{-4} M potassium cyanide at
oxygen concentrations of 0.6, 2.0 or 3.0 µM (Fig. 4). Cyanide
would have blocked the cytochrome system thereby preventing the
consumption of oxygen in its action as a terminal electron acceptor.
The lack of effect in cyanide treated cells suggests that at these
oxygen concentrations the principal pathway for energy production
is likely to be glycolysis and not electron transfer coupled to
oxidative phosphorylation. The shortening of the plateau in the

SR versus oxygen concentrations greater than 3.0 μM compared with
that seen at room temperature suggests changes in cellular biochemistry resulting either in a greater availability of oxygen above
concentrations of 3.0 μM or a greater inherent radiation sensitivity.
Whilst it is unlikely that the availability of oxygen would be
increased at 37° it is possible that changes in membrane fluidity
and fatty acid composition could change as the temperature is
increased. The full oxgyen effect was seen at 11 μM oxygen, a
value lower than that hitherto reported for mammalian cells.

In a previous paper (2) we showed that the SR versus misonidazole
concentration curve for hypoxic cells irradiated in full growth
medium or PBSA is also biphasic at room temperature, an SR of 2.0
being obtained using misonidazole at concentrations of 0.7, 1.0 or
2.0 mM. In this work the survival response of hypoxic cells was
measured over the same concentration range of misonidazole in full
growth medium at 37°C (Fig. 5). The results were similar to those
at room temperature, showing that at the higher temperature there
was no shortening of the plateau as found with oxygen.

CONCLUSIONS

This work confirms the existence of a two-component oxygen
effect on the survival of irradiated V-79-753B cells at both 37°C
and 20°C. furthermore, the two effects seem to be independent of
the NPSH status of the cells at the time of irradiation or the
presence of full medium as compared to the PBS used in earlier work.
Respiratory inhibition by cyanide also had no observable effect on
the radiation response at the oxygen concentrations tested.

REFERENCES

1. Millar, B. C., Fileden, E. M. and Steele, J. J. Int. J. Radiat.
       Biol., 36, 177, 1979.
2. Millar, B. C., Fielden, E. M. and Steele, J. J. Radiat. Res.,
       82, 478, 1980.
3. Tallentire, A., Jones, A. B. and Jacobs, G. B. Israel J.
       Chem., 10, 1185, 1972.
4. Alper, T., Moore, J. L. and Smith, P. Radiat. Res., 32, 780,
       1967.
5. Cullen, B. E. and Lansley, I. Int. J. Radiat. Biol., 1974.
6. Moore, J. L., Pritchard, J. A. V. and Smith, C. W. Int. J.
       Radiat. Biol., 22, 149, 1972.
7. Howard-Flanders, P. and Alper, T. Radiat. Res., 7, 518, 1957.
8. Kandaiya, S., Adams, G. E., Fielden, E. M. and Stratford, I.
       J. Proc. VII Symposium Microdosimetry Vol. II, 1117,
       Harwood Academic Press Ltd., Ed. J. Booz and H. G. Ebert
       1980.
9. Cooke, B. C., Fielden, E. M., Johnson, J. and Smithen, C. E.
       Radiat. Res., 65, 152, 1976.

10. Millar, B. C., Fielden, E. M. and Millar, J. L.   Int. J. Radiat.
        Biol., 33, 599, 1978.
11. Lange, N. A. (Ed.) Handbook of chemistry, p. 1093. Handbook
        Publishers Inc., Ohio, USA, 1956.
12. Cullen, B. E., Michalowski, A., Walker, H. C. and Revesz, L.
        Int. J. Radiat. Biol., 38, 525. 1980.
13. Millar, B. C., Fieldne, E. M. and Steele, J. J. Cancer Manage-
        ment Vol. V., 450, Ed. L. W. Brady, Masson Publishing
        USA Inc., 1981.
14. Kosower, M. S., Kosower, E. M. and Wirtheim, B., 1969.
15. Watts, M. E., Whillans, D. W. and Adams, G. E.   Int. J. Radiat.
        Biol. 27, 259, 1975.
16. Harris, J. W., Power, J. A. and Koch, C. J.   Radiat. Res., 64,
        270, 1975.
17. Harris, J. W., Koch, C. J., Power, J. A. and Biaglow, J. E.
        Radiat. Tes., 70, 585, 1977.

ACKNOWLEDGEMENTS

    We would like to thank Mr. J. Currant for valuable technical
assistance and the MRC/CRC for funding.

OXYGEN EFFECTS IN RADIOBIOLOGY

C. J. Koch

Radiobiology, Cross Cancer Institute

11560 University Avenue, Edmonton, Alberta, Canada T6G 1Z2

In the field of Radiobiology, (a good recent text is "Radiobiology for the Radiobiologist"; Hall, 1978) the 'Oxygen Effect'
is understood to mean the increased sensitivity of cells to damage
from ionizing radiation as the concentration of oxygen increases
from 0 to about 20,000 ppm*. Above 20,000 - 50,000 ppm the
radiation sensitivity remains about the same (see Ling et al, 1981
for one of the most accurate assessments). But oxygen affects
many aspects of cell biology and (bio) chemistry and several of
these are important in radiobiology. The purpose of this short
review is to describe several effects of oxygen pertinent to
radiobiology and to indicate problem areas where the interaction of
the Radiation Research Society and International Society for Oxygen
Transport to Tissue might be most beneficial. The reference list
is by no means comprehensive, but representative articles are listed
where appropriate.

RADIOSENSITIVITY

The enhancement of radiation damage by oxygen was first
described by Holthusen (1921) who was assessing the radiation
response of Ascaris eggs. Since then it has been demonstrated in
essentially all free-living organisms. The shapes of survival
curves are similar under aerated and hypoxic conditions, but to
achieve the same amount of killing hypoxic cells require a significantly larger radiation dose than do aerated cells (Fig. 1). The
ratio of doses given to hypoxic and aerobic cells which produce the
same surviving fractions is termed the oxygen enhancement ratio
(OER). The value of the OER is typically 2.5 → 3.0. The mechanism
of the oxygen effect is presently understood in terms of our
knowledge of basic radiation-chemistry processes. Radiation causes

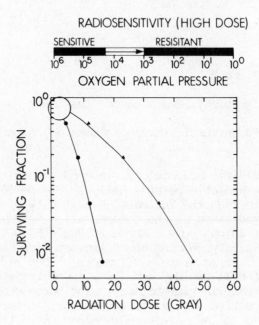

Figure 1. As the partial pressure of oxygen decreases from about
          20,000 to 1,000 ppm, cells become more radioresistant.
          For the same degree of cell killing hypoxic cells are
          given 3 times more radiation than aerobic cells. Most
          experiments in vitro are done using large single doses
          of radiation whereas most cancer therapy is effected
          using multiple small doses of radiation and the oxygen
          effect for the survival response at these low doses
          (circled area) is uncertain (see also Figures 3 and 4).

oxidative radical damage in important molecular targets (e.g. DNA
or DNA-membrane) either directly via the displacement of an electron,
or directly through the production of the hydroxyl radical (OH$^-$)
when a photon of radiation interacts with water. Subsequent
oxidation of these target radicals leads to fixation of damage,
whereas reduction leads to restitution of the original molecule
(see Chapman and Gillespie, 1981 for review - Fig. 2).

In 1953, Gray et al suggested that the oxygen concentration
in tumor cells might be critical for the successful treatment of
human cancers by ionizing radiation because the maximum dose given
is limited by damage to nearby normal tissue which is aerobic.
Since the survival of cells decreases exponentially with radiation
dose, and since production of a given degree of cell kill requires
three times the radiation dose when oxygen is absent, even a very
small percentage of radioresistant hypoxic cells could ultimately
determine the radiocurability of tumors.

The evidence for hypoxic cells in animal tumors (which grow at
a much faster rate than their human counterparts) is overwhelming
(Moulder and Rockwell, 1980, Chapman et al, in press). In human
cancer most recent evidence is indirect although O_2 measurements
in human tumors were made by Cater (1964) and Cater and Silver (1960).
Van den Brenk (1968) and Henk and Smith (1977) have reported the
results of clinical trials using hyperbaric oxygen in conjunction
with radiotherapy. Small improvements in local control were found
for patients breathing hyperbaric oxygen (compared with air) which
is evidence for the presence of hypoxic cells in these tumors.

Urtasun et al (1976) found significant increase in survival
time for patients with glioblastoma multiforme who were treated
with radiation plus metronidazole, compared with patients treated
with radiation alone. Metronidazole is an electron-affinic chemical
which, like oxygen, causes hypoxic cells to become more sensitive to
radiation damage (Adams, 1973). At present, several phase III
studies with metronidazole and another radiosensitizer, misonidazole,
are underway in Britain, the United States and Canada to evaluate
these drugs in the radiotherapy of various cancers.

In yet another type of study, Bush et al (1978) showed that
patients with carcinoma of the cervix who were anaemic during
radiotherapy (haemaglobin 12g%) had a significantly higher local
recurrence rate that those patients whose haemaglobin levels were
greater than 12g%. Furthermore, pre-therapy transfusion corrected
this discrepancy.

A serious problem arises when we try to apply our knowledge
of the oxygen effect to cancer therapy because laboratory experiments
generally are done using large single doses of radiation, while
cancer therapy usually consists of a series of very small doses

RADIATION CHEMISTRY MODEL (RCM)

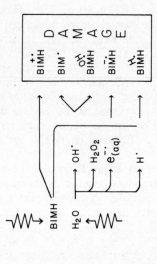

Figure 2.   Radiation acts on biologically important target molecules (BIM) either directly (resulting in loss of electron) or indirectly (from radicals produced by water radiolysis). The most important types of target damage are thought to result in the radicals BIMH$^{+\cdot}$ and BIM$\cdot$ (electron loss and hydrogen loss respectively) which are either 'fixed' by oxidation or 'repaired' by chemical reduction.

separated by 1 or 2 days. During the time between doses of radiotherapy several important processes occur, including repair of
radiation damage and re-oxygenation of the hypoxic cells (Kallman,
1968; see Withers, 1975 for review). An additional problem is that
we know little about the precise nature of the oxygen effect at
such small doses (circled area of Fig. 1). In fact there are
reports that the oxygen enhancement ratio is much reduced in this
region of the survival curve (Littbrand, 1970) although there is
considerable controversy about this (see Koch, 1975, 1979 and the
6th Gray Conference- reference in Koch, 1975). Figure 3 illustrates
the variation in survivals seen even when multiple determinations
are made and Figure 4 illustrates the range of possible oxygen
effects at low doses varying from no difference than the high dose
results to similar radiosensitivity for hypoxic and aerobic cells.

There are several important reasons for the difficulties in
determining the low-dose response with great accuracy. One is that
we are trying to determine a very small number of killed cells in
the presence of a large number of survivors. Simple statistical
fluctuations prevent the accurate determination of the number of
cells killed unless elaborate experimental methods are employed.
A second is that the oxygen dependence of cell sensitivity may
vary with the survival level and traces of oxygen may be contaminating
experimental systems. Radiation itself consumes oxygen (at the rate
of about 3 micromolar per kilorad or 10 Gray) and therefore can
remove the contaminating oxygen at higher radiation doses, but at
low doses, this contamination may strongly influence the results.
Thirdly, many of the procedures for producing hypoxia are themselves
somewhat toxic so that the hypoxic cells may already be at a disadvantage. These problems require a great deal of work. In
particular, better experimental methods are required for the
production, maintainance and measurement of low oxygen levels (Koch
1979).

REPAIR OF SUBLETHAL RADIATION DAMAGE

Sublethal radiation damage occurs as a result of the continually
increasing slope of the log survival versus dose curve (e.g. Fig. 1).
That is, each increment of dose becomes more toxic to the surviving
cells than the previous increment of dose, possibly because the
surviving cells have all been damaged to some extent by the
accumulated radiation dose (This phenomenon does not occur for most
bacterial cells which have simple exponential relationships between
survival and dose, (i.e. Survival = exp. (-k Dose)). Another way
of looking at this is that mammalian cells survive exponentially as
a function of a specific type of radiation damage, but this damage
accumulates as both a linear and quadratic function of dose. After
a given dose of radiation the surviving cells can repair the sublethal
damage, at least in part, tending to return to their original zero-
dose (decreased) sensitivity. Cells which have repaired their

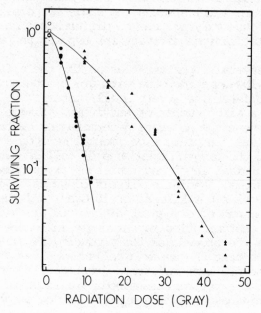

Figure 3. Actual survival curves with survival determinations
done in quadruplicate (some points in duplicate)
illustrate the statistical problems involved in
determining the radiation response at small radiation
doses.   (Koch, unpublished, using methods describing
in Koch and Biaglow, 1978).

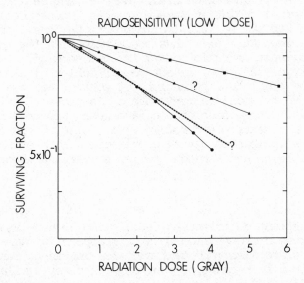

Figure 4. The range of O.E.R. reported in the literature for small
        radiation doses relevant to the clinical situations
        include:
        a)   the same OER (3) as at high doses (■ = N$_2$, ◖ = Air)
        b)   an OER which is 1 or even less (--- = N$_2$, ◕ = Air)
        or c) an intermediate value (1.5 → 2.0) (▲ = N$_2$, ● = Air).

sublethal damage are therefore less sensitive to a second dose of
radiation and exhibit a greater survival than cells which have not.
If one thinks of an experiment where cells are given two equal doses
of radiation separated by a repair interval, then the minimum
survival will be found for those cells with zero repair time (i.e.
both doses given concurrently) and the maximum for those cells with
enough time to effect as complete repair as possible (Fig. 5).

The question of whether this repair process can occur under
hypoxia was very difficult to answer because conditions of essentially
zero oxygen tension had to be maintained during and between radiation
doses. However it is now generally agreed that anoxic cells cannot
repair sub-lethal radiation damage whereas hypoxic cells with even
as little as 200 ppm O_2 (0.001 atmospheric O_2 level) can (see Koch,
1979, for review, Fig. 5). Thus one explanation for the success of
current multifraction radiotherapy is that some cells in tumors have
so little oxygen that they cannot repair sublethal damage. This
cannot be the complete explanation, of course, because it seems
likely that there would be many more cells present at intermediate
oxygen levels. These conclusions have been supported by very
difficult experiments performed in vivo. Other types of repair are
even less susceptible to oxygen deprivation (Koch et al, 1977, Koch
and Painter, 1975) and a recent review summarizes these results
(Koch, 1979).

GROWTH

Many nutrient deficiencies (e.g. amino acids - Stanners et al
1978) can cause a growth slow-down or stoppage in mammalian cells.
Other factors are also important and, for instance, many mammalian
cells stop growing because of contact with other similar cells
(Stoker, 1973).

A common finding is that the majority of tumor cells are non-
cycling, particularly in human cancer, but the reasons for the
growth stoppage are not known with certainty (Barendsen et al, 1973,
Hermens and Barendsen, 1978). A typical finding as one progresses
away from a capillary, is a decrease in the proportion of prolifer-
ating cells, although such cells are found even at the edges of
necrosis (Thomlinson and Gray, 1955, Tannock, 1968). The onset
of necrosis coincides with the calculated maximum diffusion distance
of oxygen but this assumes diffusion constants and respiration rates
similar to condition in vitro.

One finds similar results using an in vitro model of tumor
growth, the multi-cell spheroid (see Sutherland and Durand, 1976,
for review). Spheroids grow in suspension cultures to diameters of
1 mm or more, and in spheroids greater than 0.3 mm diameter one
finds 3 distinct cell types. An outer rim of cycling cells, an
annulus of non-cycling cells and an inner core of necrotic cells.

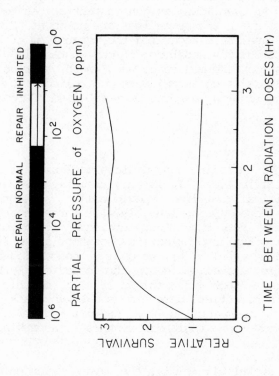

Figure 5. Repair of sublethal damage can be observed in experiments where a given dose of radiation is separated into 2 halves separated by a repair interval. Normal to low oxygen levels allow an increase in survival between split doses (upper curve) but at extremely low levels of oxygen, repair is inhibited (lower curve).

The thickness of the rim of viable cells again coincides with the oxygen diffusion distance but there is some recent evidence to suggest that other nutritional and/or waste and/or environmental factors may also play an important role (Franko and Sutherland, 1978, Freyer and Sutherland, unpublished).

In vitro results appear more clear-cut. At low cell densities cells can survive and even grow at very low oxygen concentrations – low enough to provide full protection from the oxygen-effect for cell radiosensitivity (Koch et al, 1973a, Born et al, 1976). Below about 5000 ppm, O_2 growth gradually slows until one sees either very slow growth or complete growth cessation at 50 – 200 ppm (Koch et al 1973b – Fig. 6). At even lower oxygen concentrations toxically results although here again the mechanisms are unknown. Surprisingly little data is available regarding the metabolism of hypoxic mammalian cells, particularly under conditions where cell viability and oxygen concentration were monitored, and where other nutritional an environmental factors (such as pH) were controlled. However one expects severe changes in many aspects of metabolism (Gordon et al, 1977).

CYTOTOXICITY OF DRUGS

In cancer therapy there are many different classes of drug with a broad range of specificities. It is only recently however, that the concept of specifically killing hypoxic cells by chemotherapeutic agents has been considered (Sutherland, 1974). Three general classes of drug come to mind: first; those that interfere with glycolysis or energy metabolism other than oxidative phosphorylation (e.g. glucose analogues; Song et al 1976); secondly, those which are activated by anaerobic metabolism (e.g. nitroreduction (Sutherland, 1974), dehydroascorbate (Koch and Biaglow, 1978)); and thirdly chemicals which might potentiate damage caused by the lack of the cells' ability to oxidize molecules (e.g. enzymes requiring NAD (P) +, lipid oxidation and/or prostoglandin synthesis, aspargine synthesis etc.).

In order to be useful clinically, the oxygen dependence of drug toxicity would have to complement the oxygen dependence of radiosensitivity. In addition, the drugs would have to be essentially non-toxic to aerobic tissue, particularly the stem-cell populations that are at risk for most types of chemotherapy, and would have to diffuse to the hypoxic tissue and be active at the high cell densities typical of tissue.

Clearly, these requirements will be very difficult to meet. Even with the oxygen dependence of drug toxicity there are many problems. In vitro, nitroaromatic radiation sensitizing agents like misonidazole have an extremely low Km for toxicity (Fig. 7), and so would be expected to kill only the most severely hypoxic cells

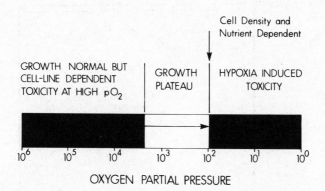

Figure 6. At normal levels of oxygen cells grow at their
maximal rate, although sometimes toxicity is seen
at very high oxygen concentrations. At oxygen
levels substantially lower than the oxygen effect
for radiosensitivity, cell growth slows or stops,
and at extremely low levels of oxygen (comparable
to the range where inhibition of repair occurs)
toxicity is found.

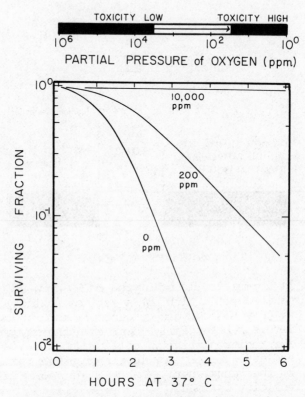

Figure 7.   Cytotoxicity of misonidazole. The cytotoxicity of
            nitro-aromatic compounds decreases dramatically with
            even very small concentration of oxygen. Figure
            adapted from Taylor and Rauth (1981) and Koch
            (unpublished).

(Taylor and Rauth, 1981). This appears to be the case in some
animal tumor models (Brown, 1977), where relatively few cells are
killed and where the tumors are known to contain chronically hypoxic
cells. Paradoxically, in multi-cell spheroids, a much greater
fraction of the total cell population is killed by these drugs
than the estimated fraction of hypoxic cells (Sutherland and Durand,
1976, Mueller-Klieser and Sutherland, 1981).

In human studies using misonidazole as a hypoxic cell radiosensitizer, the maximum concentration of drug that can be used in
a multi-fraction regimen is limited to 100 M by nervous system
toxicity (Urtasun et al, 1978). As yet no appropriate model exists
for this presumably aerobic toxicity, and the concentration of drug
(100 M) is about 50 times less than that required for useful hypoxic
tumor-cell cytotoxicity.

A similar very low Km has been found for the toxicity of glucose-
analogues like 2 deoxy-glucose (Koch, unpublished) so one would not
expect these drugs to be an effective chemotherapy agent against
hypoxic cells. One compound, dehydroascorbate, has been found to
have a high Km for toxicity (Koch and Biaglow, 1978) but the toxicity
also extends to aerobic cells. Unfortunately, no hypoxic cell
toxicity could be demonstrated for this drug in vivo (Koch, unpublished), even at concentrations which would be expected to cause
alloxan-type diabetes.

FUTURE WORK

If one accepts the premise that hypoxic cells pose a problem
in the cure of cancer by radiotherapy there are many questions of
immediate interest:
    1.   What are the principal nutrient deficiencies and/or waste
products which cause the development of viable hypoxic cells?
    2.   Can hypoxic cells adapt to these environments by reducing
their oxygen consumption rate?
    3.   Are there unique metabolic weaknesses of these cells which
could be exploited by appropriate chemotherapy?
    4.   What is the mechanism of re-oxygenation between fractions
of radiation?
    5.   Can we inhibit oxygen consumption by relatively non-toxic
means?
    6.   Can we monitor the proportion of hypoxic cells in a tumor
during a course of radiotherapy and use this information to
successfully alter the schedule of treatments?

Although several of these questions appear answerable by in
vitro experiments there remains the problem of relevance to the
in vivo situation. In particular, it is usually impossible to do
any long term experiments at cell densities even approaching those
found in vivo (e.g. 10^9 cells/cc). One exception is the development

of the multi-cell spheroid model, which achieves tissue-like densities
in the discrete spheroids, but at an average cell density in the
medium which is quite low (Sutherland and Durand, 1976).

In a series of recent experiments Mueller-Klieser and Sutherland
(submitted 1981) have measured the oxygen tension profiles through
these spheroids, using exceptionally fine electrodes (Whalen et al
1973). Their elegant experimental set-up has demonstrated symmetrical
O_2 tension profiles as the electrode passes through a spheroid and
the results often show a central plateau of non-zero oxygen level
in spheroids which have large necrotic centers. Thus we see necrosis
without hypoxia, but in addition, oxygen levels substantially higher
than would be expected from diffusion constants and cellular respiration rates determined with cell suspensions in vitro (Froese,
1962).

Other tantalizing results from experiments in vitro have hinted
at the ability of cells to adapt to unfavorable environments by
lowering oxygen consumption rates (Vail and Glinos, 1974, Koch and
Biaglow, 1978, Fig. 8) but no general control mechanisms are yet
known which could substantially change the rate of respiration.
It is certainly clear that many cells can survive and even grow
despite drastically decreased oxygen supplies. In three cell lines
tested, there was almost no growth inhibition by 2 mM KCN,
despite the fact that as little as 0.5 mM KCN reduces respiration by
more than 95% (Fig. 9). It is important to continue the search for
inhibitors of cell respiration which are less toxic in vivo, since
this could lead to rapid re-oxygenation of hypoxic tumor cells during
each fraction of a course of radiotherapy which might cause a great
increase in tumor radiocurability. One such inhibitor is hyperthermia, which has been shown to increase both blood flow and pO_2
in several tissues including tumor (Bicher et al, 1980).

A major problem with respiration rate experiments in vitro is
the use of equipment that is toxic to the cells (e.g. slow homo-
genzation of fragile cells by stirring bars, cell densities which
allow nutrient depletion in minutes, etc. - see also Koch and Biaglow
1978). Often one finds that such damaged cells respond very differ-
ently to drugs and environmental conditions than do cells held under
conditions optimized for growth and high viability. This problem
is somewhat analogous to differences seen in the use of coupled vs
uncoupled mitochondria. An improved design of a sealable container
for mammalian cell respiration experiments (Koch and Biaglow, 1978)
is shown in Fig. 10.

The importance of testing in vivo, the concepts derived from
in vitro work cannot be overemphasized, but at present, the oxygen
measurement technology cannot provide non-invasive measurements with
good resolution, particularly at large distances from the skin. A
new development has been the demonstration that drugs like

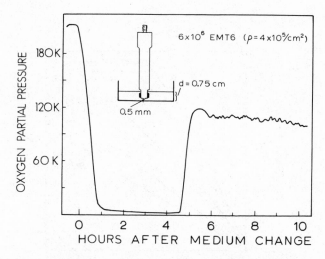

Figure 8. Confluent cells attached to the surface of a flat glass dish seem to adapt to the diffusion barrier imposed by a large volume of medium. Although the oxygen partial pressure drops to extremely low levels just after fresh medium is added to the culture, the oxygen tension subsequently rises to a level much higher than expected if the cells were consuming oxygen at the normal rate (Koch and Biaglow, 1978).

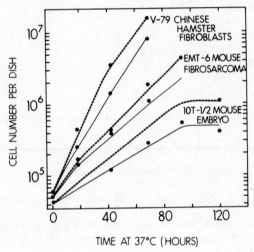

Figure 9. All cell lines tested to date grow at almost the normal
          rate (---) in the present of 2.0 mM KCN (——). From
          parallel long term experiments using the apparatus of
          Fig. 10, it is known that the cellular oxygen consumption
          rate is continuously reduced by greater than 95% with
          even 0.5 mM KCN.

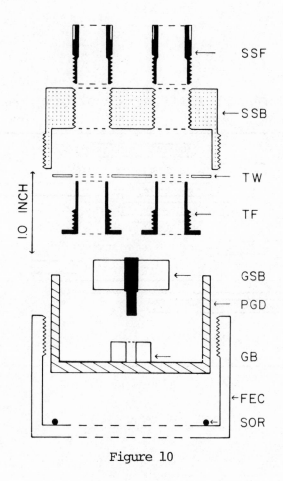

Figure 10

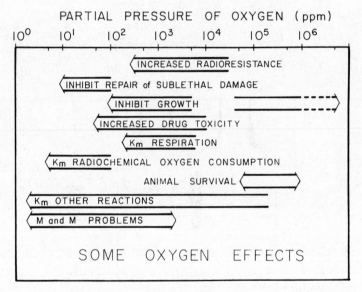

Figure 11

misonidazole bind specifically to molecules in hypoxic cells, presumably through anaerobic metabolism (Chapman et al, 1981). Present
work is focused on the relationships between drug binding and
cytotoxicity, drug binding and degree of hypoxia, and the development
of a gamma-emitting analogue which could be used to identify hypoxic
cells using nuclear medicine techniques. Other drugs and reaction
types may also be useful in this type of assay.

In summary, the primary goal in radiobiological research
relating to oxygen, as in other areas involving oxygen effects and
transport, is the continued development of new methods to measure
and control oxygen concentrations both in vivo and in vitro. Oxygen
concentration is an important variable affecting many areas of
interest to radiobiology and to other fields as well (Fig. 11).

*Oxygen concentrations throughout this paper are given in terms of
parts per million partial pressure. For medium equilibrated with
air at 37°C and one atmosphere the following measures are equivalent:

O_2 in air = 21% = 210,000 ppm = 159 mm Hg = 21.2 kPa = 220 µM =
$7^{.0}$ ppm (weight) = 0.49 cc/100 mls.

REFERENCES

1. Adams, G. E. Chemical radiosensitization of hypoxic cells.
      Brit. Med. Bull., 29: 48-53, 1973.
2. Barendsen, G. W., Roelse, H., Hermens, A. F., Madhuizen, H. T.,
      van Peperyul, H. A., and Rutgers, D. H. Clonogenic
      capacity of proliferating and nonproliferating cells of
      a transplantable rat rhabdomyosarcoma in relation to its
      radiosensitivity. J. Natl. Cancer Inst. 51: 1521-1526,
      1973.
3. Bicher, H. I., Hetzel, F. W., Sandhu, T. S., Frinak, S.,
      Vaupel, P., O'Hara, M. D. and O'Brien, T. Effects of
      Hyperthermia on normal and tumor microenvironment. Radio-
      logy 137, 523-530, 1980.
4. Born, R., Hug, O. and Trott, K. R. The effect of prolonged
      hypoxia on growth and viability of Chinese hamster cells.
      Int. J. Radiat. Oncol. Biol. Physics 1: 687-697, 1976.
5. Brown, J. M., Cytotoxic effects of the hypoxic cell radio-
      sensitizer Ro-07-0582 to tumor cells in vivo. Radiat.
      Res. 72: 469-486, 1977.
6. Bush, R. S., Jenkin, R. D. T., Allt, W. E. C., Beale, F. A.,
      Bean, H., Demko, A. J. and Pringle, J. F. Definitive
      evidence for hypoxic cells influencing cure in cancer
      therapy. Brit. J. Cancer, 37: Suppl. iii, 302-306, 1978.
7. Cater, D. B. Oxygen tension in neoplastic tissues. Tumori,
      50: 435-444, 1964.
8. Cater, D. B., and Silver, I. A. Quantitative measurements of
      oxygen tension in normal tissues and in the tumors of

patients before and after radiotherapy. Acta Radio., 53: 233-256, 1960.

9. Chapman, J. D., and Gillespie, C. J. Radiation induced events and their timescale in mammalian cells. In "Advances in Radiation Biology" Academic Press (In Press).

10. Chapman, J. D., Franko, A. J. and Sharplin, J. A marker for hypoxic cells in tumors with potential clincial applicability. Br. J. Cancer 43: 546-550, 1981.

11. Chapman, J. D., Franko, A. J. and Koch, C. J. The fraction of hypoxic clonogenic cells in tumor populations. In "Proceedings of 2nd Rome International Symposium - Biological Bases and Clincical Implications of Tumor Radioresistance (Eds. C. Nervi, G. Arcangeli, and F. Mauro) (In Press).

12. Franko, A. J. and Sutherland, R. M. The rate of death of hypoxic cells in multi cell spheroids. Radit. Res. 76: 561-572, 1978.

13. Froese, G. The respiration of ascites tumor cells at low oxygen concentrations. Biochem. Biophys. Acta. 57: 509-519, 1962.

14. Gordon, G. B., Barcza, M. A., and Bush, M. E. Lipid accumulation in hypoxic tissue culture cells. Am. J. Pathology 88: 663-678, 1977.

15. Gray, L. H., Conger, A. D., Ebert, M., Hornsey, S. and Scott, O. C. A., Concentration of oxygen dissolved in tissues at time of irradiation as a factor in radiotherapy. Brit. J. Radiol., 26: 638-648, 1953.

16. Hall, E. J. Radiobiology for the RAdiobiologist (2nd ed) Harper and Row Maryland, 1978.

17. Henk, J. M., and Smith, C. W. Radiotherapy and hyperbaric oxygen in head and neck cancer: Interim report of second clinical trial. Lancet, 2: 104, 1977.

18. Hermens, A. F. and Barendsen, G. W., The proliferative status and clonogenic capacity of tumor cells in a transplantable rhabdomyosarcoma of the rat before and after irradiation with 800 rad x-rays. Cell Tissue Kinet., 11: 83-100, 1978.

19. Holthusen, H. Bertrage zur biologie der strahlenwirkung. Pfluger's Archiv fur die Gesante Physiologie 187: 1-24, 1921.

20. Kallman, R. F., Repopulation and reoxygenation as factors contributing to the effectiveness of fractionated radiotherapy. Front. Radiat. Ther. Oncol., 3: 96-108, 1968.

21. Koch, C. J. Measurement of very low oxygen tensions in liquids: Does the extrapolation number for mammalian cells decrease after x-irradiation under anoxic conditions. In: Cell survival after low doses of radiation, Proc. 6th Gray Conf., Sept. '74, Ed. T. Alper, Institute of Physics and John Wiley and Sons. 167-171, 1975.

22. Koch, C. J. The effect of oxygen on the repair of radiation damage by cells and Tissues. In: Advances in Radiation

Biology 8: 273-315, 1979, (J. T. Lett and H. Alder, eds)
Academic Press, New York.

23. Koch, C. J. and Biaglow, J. E. Toxicity, Radiation Sensitivity
modification and metabolic effects of dehydroascorbate and
ascorbate in mammalian cells. J. Cell. Phys. 94: 299-
306, 1978.

24. Koch, C. J., and Biaglow, J. E. Respiration of mammalian cells
at low concentrations of oxygen: 1. Effect of hypoxic-cell
radiosensitizing drugs. Br. J. Cancer 37: Suppl. III,
163-167, 1978.

25. Koch, C. J. and Painter, R. B., The effect of extreme hypoxia
on the repair of DNA Single-Strand-Breaks in mammalian
cells. Radiat. Res. 64: 256-269, 1975.

26. Koch, C. J., Kruuv, J. and Frey, H. E. The effect of hypoxia
on the generation time of mammalian cells. Radiat. Res.
53: 43-480, 1973.

27. Koch, C. J., Men es, J. J. and Harris, J. W. The effect of
extreme hypoxia and glucose on the repair of potentially
lethal and sublethal radiation damage by mammalian cells.
Radiat. Res. 70: 542, 1977.

28. Koch, C. J., Kruuv, J., Frey, H. E. and Snyder, Ra. A. Plateau
phase in growth induced by hypoxia. Int. J. Radiat. Biol.
23: 67-74, 1973.

29. Ling, C. C., Michaels, H. B., Gerweck, L. E., Epp, E. R. and
Peterson, E. C. Oxygen Sensitization of Mammalian Cells
under different irradiation conditions. Radiat. Res.
86: 325-340, 1981.

30. Littbrand, B. Survival characteristics of mammalian cell lines
after single or multiple exposures to Roentgen radiation
under oxic or anoxic conditions. Acta Radiologica. Ther.
Phys. Biol. 9: 257-281, 1970.

31. Moulder, J. E., and Rockwell, S. C., Survey of published data
on the hypoxic fractions of solid rodent tumors. Radiat.
Res., 83, 376, 1980.

32. Mueller-Klieser, W. F. and Sutherland, R. M. Oxygen tensions
in multicell spheroids of two cell lines at different
stages of growth. Submitted 1981.

33. Song, C. W., Clement, J. J. and Levitt, S. H. Preferential
cytotoxicity of 5-thio-D-glucose against Hypoxic tumor
cells. J. Natl. Cancer Inst. 57: 603, 1976.

34. Stanners, C. P., Wightman, T. M. and Harkins, J. L. Effect of
extreme amino acid starvation on the protein synthetic
machinery of CHO cells. J. Cellular Physiology 95: 125-
138, 1978.

35. Stoker, M. G. P., Role of diffusion boundary layer in contact
inhibition of growth. Nature 246: 200-203, 1973.

36. Sutherland, R. M. Selective chemotherapy of noncycling cells
in an in vitro tumor model. Cancer Res. 34: 3501-3503,
1974.

37. Sutherland, R. M. and Durand, R. E. Radiation Response of

multicell spheroids - an in vitro tumor model. Curr. Top.
Radiat. Res. Q. 11: 87-139, 1976.
38. Tannock, I. F. The relation between cell proliferatin and the
    vascular system in a transplanted mouse mammary tumor.
    Brit. J. Cancer, 22: 258-273, 1968.
39. Taylor, Y. C. and Rauth, A. M. Oxygen tension, cellular
    respiration and redox states as variable influencing the
    cytotoxicity of the radiosensitizer misonidazole. Radiat.
    Res. In Press, 1981.
40. Thomlinson, R. H. and Gray, L. H. The histological structure
    of some human lung cancers and the possible implications
    for radiotherapy. Br. J. Cancer 9: 539-549, 1955.
41. Urtasun, R. C., Band, P., Chapman, J. D., Feldstein, M. L.,
    Mielke, B., and Fryer, C. Radiation and high-dose
    metronidazole in supratentorial glioblastomas. New Eng.
    J. Med., 294: 1364-1367, 1976.
42. Urtasun, R. C., Chapman, J. D., Feldstein, M. L. Band, R. P.,
    Rabin, H. E., Wilson, A. F., Marynowski, B., Starreveld,
    A., and Shmitka, T., Peripheral neuropathy related to
    misonidazole: Incidence and Pathology. Br. J. Cancer 37
    (Suppl III) 271-275, 1978.
43. Vail, J. M. and Glinos, A. D. Density dependent regulation of
    growth in L-cell suspension cultures V. Adaptive and
    nonadaptive respiratory decline. Cell. Physiology 83:
    425-436, 1974.
44. Van den Brenk, H. A. Hyperbaric oxygen in radiation therapy.
    An investigation of dose-effect relationships. Am. J.
    Roentgen. 102, 8, 1968
45. Whalen, W. J., Nair, P., and Granfield, R. A. Measurements
    of oxygen tension in tissues with a micro oxygen electrode.
    Microvasc. Res. 5: 254, 1973.
46. Withers, H. R. The 4 R's of Radiotherapy In: Advances in
    Radiation Biology 5: 241-271, 1975 (J. Lett and H. Adler,
    eds.) Academic Press, New York.

LOCAL IONIZING RADIATION WITH AND WITHOUT MICROWAVE INDUCED

HYPERTHERMIA IN SUPERFICIAL MALIGNANT TUMORS IN BRAIN

C.E. Lindholm, E. Kjellen, T. Landberg, C. Mercke,
P. Nilsson, and B. Persson

Lund and Malmo University Hospitals
Sweden

In order to generate local hyperthermia in superficial malignant tumor in man a computerized system using a 2 450 MHz microwave generator connected to a circular direct contact applicator (diameter 90 mm) has been constructed. The automatic control system uses a pulsed irradiation technique and reads the tumor and normal tissue temperature via thermistor probes. The microcomputer regulates the output power of the microwave generator and maintains the preset temperature in the centre of the tumor with a maximum temperature ripple of $\pm 0.3^{\circ}C$. Superficial tumors of less than 7 cm diameter and of less than 3 cm depth have been accepted for treatment. The ionizing radiation beams have been conventional X-ray, electrons and [137] Cs gama rays. Ionizing radiation has been given with 3.00 Gy for 10 fractions (5 fractions per week) to a total dose of 30.0 Gy. The hyperthermial level has been $42.5^{\circ}C - 43.5^{\circ}C + 0.3^{\circ}C$ during 45 minutes once or twice a week for 2 weeks with at least 72 hours between each hyperthermia treatment. In case of more than one superficial tumor in the same patient a comparison between the effect of radiation alone, hyperthermia alone and the combination of those two modalities has been performed according to a pre-scribed protocol. The time gap between radiation and hyperthermia has been 1 or 4 hours in different schedules in order to compare the effect on normal tissue and tumor according to timing and fraction.

Eleven patients have started treatment since the first of August, 1980; 9 have completed the treatment, 4 have had more than one superficial lesion, allowing for comparison of the effect of different treatment modalities. More rapid and pronounced and also

145

more lasting tumor regressions were found in tumors treated with
the combination of the two modalities compared to tumors treated
with only radiotherapy or hyperthermia alone.

OXYGEN, HYDROGEN DONORS AND RADIATION RESPONSE

John E. Biaglow, Associate Professor

Radiation Biochemistry, School of Medicine

Case Western Reserve University, Cleveland, Ohio 44106

THE OXYGEN EFFECT WITH CELLS

No other chemical has been as widely studied as oxygen and
yet continues to be such an intensive subject of study as a sensitizer
of mammalian cells (Alpher, 1979; Elkind and Sinclair, 1965; Puch
and Marcus, 1956; Hall, 1978; Groesch and Hopwood, 1979). The
early studies of Gray et al., 1958, Fig. 1, indicate that as the
oxygen concentration is lowered there is a corresponding decrease
in the radiation response of cells. The relative radiosensitivity
of cells increases rapidly between 0 and 0.3% oxygen. Further
increases occur until approximately 30 mm oxygen after which
additional increases are very small. The OER (Oxygen Enhancement
Ratio), or relative radiosensitivity, varies between 2 and 3.5 for
the majority of cells (Hall, 1978). Oxygen has been studied as a
sensitizer because of the problem thought to occur in vitro with
human tumors. Human tumor cells outgrow their blood supply resulting
in a decreased availabiltiy of oxygen and resulting in hypoxic and
anoxic tumor areas which may exhibit a decreased radiation response.
The chief cause of the oxygen effect in vivo is due to the consumption
of oxygen by the tumor cells. The metabolic utilization of oxygen
decreased the distance to which it may penetrate in the cells more
distant from the capillaries. Unlike the physiological situation,
most experiments are performed in vitro with cells that have been
equilibrated with a nitrogen-carbon dioxide gas mixture for a
period of time that insures the depletion of the dissolved oxygen.
These procedures are laborious and require special equipment. A
simpler way of demonstrating the oxygen effect is to concentrate
cells into a dense suspension approaching in vivo cell densities.
We have found that cells under these conditions exhaust their supply
of oxygen within minutes (Fig. 2) and may be immediately irradiated,

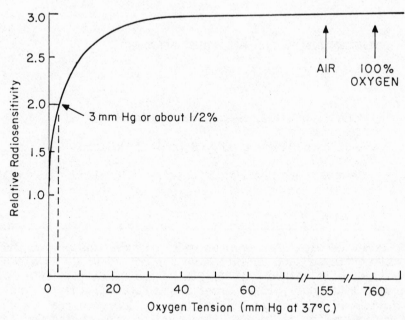

Figure 1.   Illustration of the dependence of radiosensitivity on
            oxygen concentration. If the radiosensitivity under
            anoxic conditions is arbitrarily assigned a value of unity,
            the radiosensitivity is about 3 under well-oxygenated
            conditions. Most of this change of sensitivity occurs
            as the oxygen concentration increases from zero to 30 mm
            of mercury. A further increase of oxygen content to the
            level characteristic of air, or even pure oxygen at high
            pressure, has little further effect. A sensitivity half-
            way between anoxia and full oxygenation occurs at a partial
            pressure of oxygen of about 3 mm, which corresponds to
            about 0.5%. This diagram is idealized and does not
            represent any specific experimental data. Experiments
            have been performed with yeast, bacteria, and mammalian
            cells in culture; the results conform to the general
            conclusions summarized above.

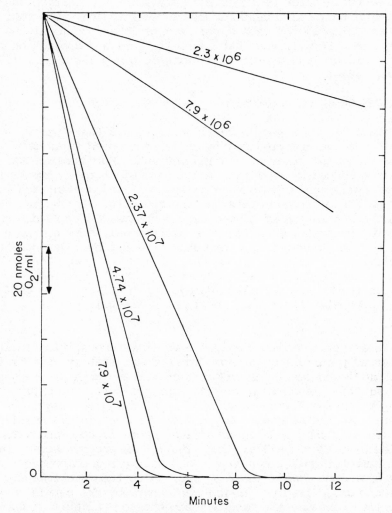

Figure 2   The effect of different densities of cells on the rate
of depletion of oxygen in a sealed container.   The
disappearance of oxygen was monitored with a Clark oxygen
electrode.   The cells were incubated at 37°C in 20 mM
HEPES buffered physiological saline, pH 7.4.

diluted and plated for survival assays.

In Fig. 3 we have determined the radiation response of this
type of dense cell suspension and have compared it to the radiation
response obtained for cells at the same density but irradiated at
zero degree to inhibit cellular oxygen utilization. The ratio of
D_O values (slopes) for each curve results in a dose modifying factor
of 3.3. The OER will vary between cell lines and depends on the
previous history and growth conditions of the cells (Hall, 1978;
Biaglow, 1981).

MECHANISMS OF OXYGEN EFFECT

Howard Flanders and Moore (1958) proposed that two types of
radiation damage are produced in cells, one which is oxygen
dependent and the other oxygen independent. For example DNA
radicals produced by radiation would be subject to a competitive
chemical challenge, with oxygen on the one hand and intracellular
donors on the other competing for the radicals. In the absence of
oxygen the first type of oxygen dependent damage may revert chemically
to a harmless state, possibly chemically repaired by hydrogen
donation from SH-containing compounds or other hydrogen-donating
molecules:

$$R\cdot + XSH \longrightarrow RH + \cdot XS$$

If oxygen reacts the so-called damage may be fixed. The cell is
unable to repair itself thus resulting in lethality:

$$R\cdot + O_2 \longrightarrow RO_2^{\overset{\bullet}{-}}$$

There is as yet, no direct evidence for this competition in irradiated
cellular systems, although there is no doubt that it applies in
simple model systems. The competition between chemical repair and
oxygen fixation leads to a working hypothesis for the oxygen effect.
This approach was further developed by studying the reactions of
suspected DNA radicals with oxygen, electron affinic sensitizers
and sulfhydryl compounds in irradiated bacteriophage and with
purified DNA (Alpher, 1979; Ward, 1957). A reaction scheme based
on the competition between oxygen and sulfhydryl compounds for the
oxygen dependent damage was proposed. With the development of
alkaline sucrose gradient techniques other workers carried out
experiments to study the oxygen dependence on radiation-induced
single strand breaks. Strand breakage was enhanced in the presence
of oxygen by a factor of 2 to 3 (Alper, 1979). Others (Painter,
et al., 1980; Roots and Okada, 1975) studied DNA strand breakage
efficiency as a function of oxygen concentration and concluded that
the oxygen effects on strand breakage are similar to those of the
radiation killing. These results were interpreted as supporting
the viewpoint that the radiation target associated with reproductive
death by the oxygen effects is DNA. Agreement on this subject that
other target sites such as the membrane may be important in radiation-induced cellular inactivation, particularly in vivo with lung

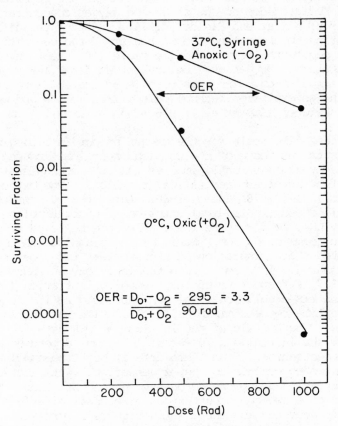

Figure 3. The effect of metabolically produced hypoxia on the radiation response in dense suspensions of Chinese hamster ovary cells. In the top curve the 2×10^8 CHO cells/ml in 0.02 M HEPES buffered media were drawn up into a glass syringe, immediately radiated, at 37°C, diluted and assayed for clonogenic survival. In the lower curve the same density of cells was spread as a layer of cells on the surface of a T30 flask, gassed with humidified CO_2 and irradiated at 0°C, diluted and assayed for colony forming ability.

and heart tissue (Okada, 1969).

Despite considerable research in past years, the basic mechanism
by which oxygen sensitizes cells to the action of radiation is still
not completely understood. For example there are reported deviations
from the predicted dependence of OER on oxygen concentration (Epp,
et al., 1976; Millar and Fielden, 1979). Part of the difficulty
in attempting to understand the mechanism of radiosensitization by
oxygen is due to the very fast time scale (10^{-3} sec) involved in
these processes. Oxygen must be present at least $1-2 \times 10^{-3}$ sec
prior to irradiation. This has been demonstrated using rapid mixing
systems, a gas explosion method, pulsed irradiation and mechanical
mixing techniques (Epp et al., 1976 ; Adams, 1980).

The fast time scale for the oxygen effect in biological systems,
combined with knowledge of the chemical reactions induced by radiation
of aqueous systems, strongly implies that the mechanism for the
oxygen effect involves free radical reactions. The oxygen fixation
hypothesis (Hall, 1978; Adams, 1980) states that O_2 reacts with
radiation-induced free radical sites on the target molecules,
presumably DNA, to form peroxides, which are believed to be non-
repairable forms of damage. Rapid mixing technique (Adams, 1980)
demonstrated that irradiation at the shortest time possible after
mixing, about 4×10^{-3} sec., resulted in an oxygen enhancement
ratio of 1.7, irrespective of the oxygen concentration (from 1 to
50%) in the mixed solution. The OER increased to its full value of
2.8 as the time between mixing and irradiation was increased to 4
$\times 10^{-2}$ sec. The profile of the increase of OER as a function of
time after the initial 4×10^{-3} sec. level was dependent on the
oxygen concentration. From these data it might be concluded that
there are two components to the oxygen effect, with the slower
one demonstrating a dependence on oxygen concentration. The
hypothesis of a two-component oxygen or sensitizer effect has not
been widely accepted and there is much current work in this area.

HYPOXIC CELL RADIOSENSITIZING DRUGS (OXYGEN MIMICKING)

In the last decade there has been rapid development in the
field of specific radiosensitizers for hypoxic cells, due largely
to the work of numerous chemists and radiobiologists (Adams, 1980)
who defined the desirable criteria for these agents and then set
out to select and design appropriate compounds. Most of the
initial work was performed with cultured cells (Adams, 1978).
Basically there was an attempt to develop drugs that would not be
metabolized as rapidly as oxygen, yet would be oxygen-mimicking
and possibly of use for in vivo sensitizing of hypoxic tumor cells.
The electron affinic, hypoxic cell radiosensitizing drugs all
contain an aromatic ring and a nitro (NO_2) group, which appears to
be the critical structural feature. Sensitizer studies to date
include nitrobenzenes, nitrofurans, nitroimidazoles, nitropyrroles

and nitropyrazoles (Fowler, et al, 1976). The most important nitro compounds (Fig. 4) so far studied are the nitroimidazoles Metronidazole (Flagyl) and Misonidazole. In Figure 5 are seen the effects of Misonidazole on hypoxic cells. There is a small effect with 1 mM, however, the response is greatly improved but not as good as O_2 when the concentration is increased to 10 mM. There is no effect of sensitization in the presence of oxygen. The effect of medium containing dissolved oxygen, (0.2 mM) is also seen. Various nitro aromatic compounds sensitize hypoxic cells to x-rays by increasing the slope of the survival curve; they do not affect the shoulder except under conditions of prolonged contact prior to irradiation (Hall and Biaglow, 1977). Demonstration of the radio-sensitizing ability of a compound in vitro is no guarantee of favorable results in vivo, since there may be biochemical, physiological or pharmacological complexities involved in vivo which might interfer with sensitizer action. For example, alterations in cellular biochemicals (Biaglow, 1981) as well as effects on cellular oxygen utilization (Biaglow, 1980) may alter the effectiveness of the agents in vivo (see Oxygen Sparing Drugs).

Unfortunately, except for a few isolated cases, the basic studies on the mechanism of action of many of these compounds have been superseded in an attempt to find drugs that will be clinically valuable. With practicality as a guideline, the nitro-imidazoles are being used for studies with humans. Metronidazole and Misonidazole (Ro-07-0582) are undergoing clinical trials in several cancer centers. At this time, studies are being carried out to determine appropriate dose and fractionation schemes for both drugs and radiation. This would result in therapeutic gain due to radiosensitization in selected tumor sites, e.g. brain, without the complication of neurotoxicity observed during the early stages of testing these compounds. Another limitation of these drugs is the effective concentration that must be reached within the tumor to achieve an observable radiosensitization. These concentrations lie in the range of 0.5 to 1 mM, which produces a dose modifying factor of 1.2 to 1.7. Another difficulty is that clinicians use low radiation doses in order to prevent mistakes; consequently the improvement in the actual radiation response in humans is at present marginal (Brady, 1980).

MECHANISM OF ACTION OF HYPOXIC CELL RADIOSENSITIZERS

There is general agreement that the electron-affinic sensitizers mimic the action of oxygen at the level of DNA (Adams, 1979). These contentions are supported by the facts that these sensitizers have no radiation effect on aerated cells, and the ability to sensitize is closely correlated with the one-electron reduction potential, a measure of electron affinity determined by pulse radiolysis (Adams, 1980). Oxygen has the highest one-electron reduction potential and is the most effective radiosensitizer.

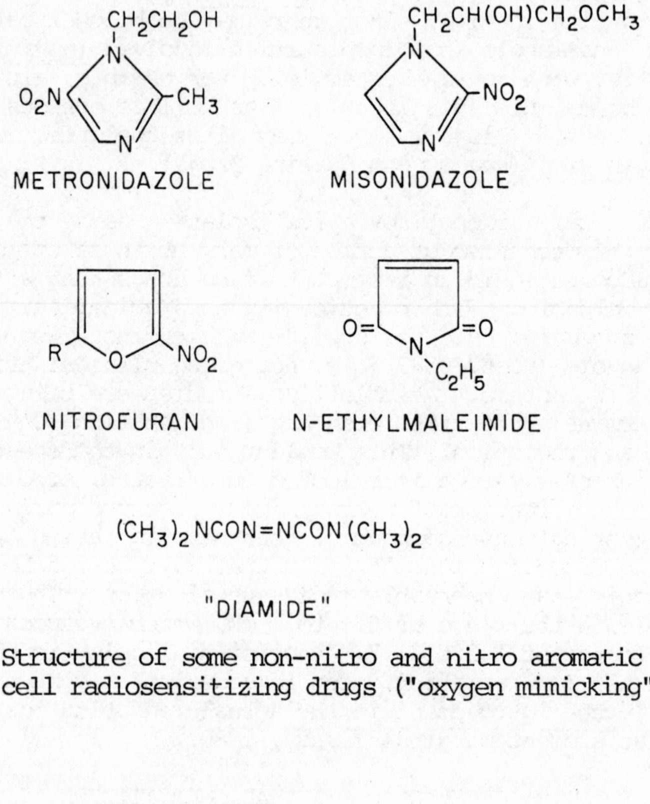

CH$_2$CH$_2$OH

O$_2$N   CH$_3$

METRONIDAZOLE

CH$_2$CH(OH)CH$_2$OCH$_3$

NO$_2$

MISONIDAZOLE

R   O   NO$_2$

NITROFURAN

O= =O

N

C$_2$H$_5$

N-ETHYLMALEIMIDE

(CH$_3$)$_2$NCON=NCON(CH$_3$)$_2$

"DIAMIDE"

Figure 4.   Structure of some non-nitro and nitro aromatic hypoxic cell radiosensitizing drugs ("oxygen mimicking").

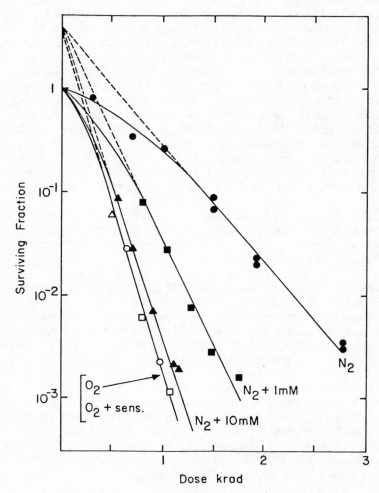

Figure 5. The effect of Misonidazole on the radiation response of hypoxic Chinese hamster ovary cells (Adams, 1979).

The electron affinity parameter is obviously important, but other
variables have been investigated. Since penetration of the sensitizer
to hypoxic cells of a tumor is of fundamental importance for effectiveness in vivo, it is reasoned that high solubility in lipids might
be a desirable feature in enhancing the diffusion of the drug.
Studies of the octanol:water partition coefficient of sensitizers
were therefore conducted (Brady, 1980). It was found that there
is no correlation between sensitizer effectiveness and lipophilicity.
Side effects such as neurotoxicity may be enhanced if the drug
partitions itself in high lipid containing tissue such as brain
(Brady, 1980). Additional studies have demonstrated that nitro
compounds are far from inert and that upon addition to cells they
profoundly alter cellular electron transfer processes involving
cellular respiration (Biaglow, 1980, 1981a). Intracellular levels
of reduced species such as NAD(P)H and glutathione are also
affected (Biaglow, 1981a). The effect of the hypoxic cell radiosensitizing drug Misonidazole on cellular glutathione (Fig. 6) and
protein thiols has been demonstrated and may be the reason that
this drug shows an enhanced radiation response when cells are
preincubated with the drug for prolonged periods (Fig. 5).

Cells also show an enhanced radiation response when pretreated
with Misonidazole alone, washed and then irradiated under hypoxic
conditions. However, cells are more sensitive in the presence of
Misonidazole (Biaglow, 1981a).

Other studies have shown that if the thiols are removed by
the sulfhydryl oxidizing agent Diamide there is a synergistic effect
on the radiation response that is greater than that obtainable
by either agent alone (Biaglow, 1981). Harris and Power, 1973, .
reported a lower survival at both 800 and 1200 rads for anoxic cells
irradiated in the presence of Diamide and Nifuroxime (a nitrofuran)
than was observed for either sensitizer alone. Similarly, Chapman
et al (1973) showed that Diamide plus NF-269, another nitrofuran,
sensitized to a greater degree than that of either agent alone, and
more than oxygen. Watts et al (1975) found that the combination of
Diamide and Misonidazole was more effective than each individual
(Fig. 7). Diamide and Misonidazole together sensitized to a
greater extent than oxygen and gave results similar to the effect
found for Diamide in the presence of oxygen.

HYDROGEN DONORS AND CHEMICAL REPAIR OF RADIATION DAMAGE

The pretreatment effects with Misonidazole (Hall and Biaglow,
1977) and the combination studies with the thiol oxidant Diamide
(Harris and Power, 1973; Chapman, 1973) suggest that endogenous
reducing species are important in the overall mechanism of radiation
damage and repair. As mentioned previously, the reaction of the
DNA radicals with hydrogen donor or reducing substrates will result
in chemical repair of the radiation damage. Some of the intra-

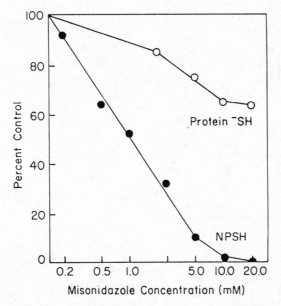

Figure 6. The effect of Misonidazole on the nonprotein and the
protein thiol content of Ehrlich ascites tumor cells.
Cells (10^7/ml) were inclubated anaerobically in 0.05 M
PBS and 10 mM glucose at 37°C, pH 7.3. Thiol determinations were performed 15 min after anaerobic conditions
had been achieved (Varnes et al, 1980).

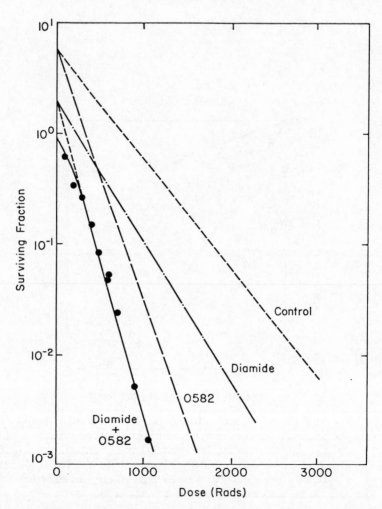

Figure 7.   Sensitization of V79-GL 1 cells to 250 kVp x-rays by
100 μM Diamide plus 5 mM Ro-07-0582 (Misonidazole)
in deoxygenated MEM + 15% serum.   The broken lines show
the survival observed for the same concentrations of
Diamide or Misonidazole independently as well as for
the no-drug control (Watts et al, 1975).

cellular hydrogen donors that are capable of reacting with radicals
are reduced flavins, reduced pyridine nucleotides, ascorbate and
thiols. The largest concentration of intracellular reducing materials
consists of protein thiols, the most important low molecular non-
protein thiol being glutathione. Intracellular glutathione is
believed to be an important hydrogen donor under anaerobic conditions
for repair of radiation induced radicals in DNA. However, it cannot
compete effectively with oxygen in air at low cell densities
because the rate of reaction of oxygen with DNA radicals is at
least an order of magnitude greater than the reaction rate with
thiols (Greenstock and Dunlop, 1975). In addition, under the
experimental conditions used for studies on the radiation response
of cells, the cell density is usually quite low: 10,000 or less.
If we assume that there is 5 nmoles NPSH/10^9 cells than 10,000 cells
would contribute approximately 5 x 10^{-11} moles of NPSH. This compares
to an oxygen tension near 2 x 10^{-7}M. Even if we allow for a factor
of 10 for the contribution of the protein thiols as radioprotectors
the thiol concentration is still only 5 x 10^{-10}M. Oxygen would be
in great excess compared to either protein or nonprotein thiols.

CELLULAR THIOLS AND RADIATION RESPONSE

There have been many attempts to remove the cellular endogenous
radioprotecting species with agents such as N-ethylmaleimide (NEM)
(Sinclair, 1975: Harris and power, 1973). In the case of Diamide
(Biaglow and Nygaard, 1973) there is a spontaneous chemical reaction
with the cellular non-protein thiols as well as with cellular reduced
pyridine nucleotides. This reaction can be utilized to an advantage
during hypoxic conditions and has been found to increase the radiation
response (Harris and Power, 1973). Diamide (Fig. 8) was found to
radiosensitize hypoxic Chinese hamster cells by decreasing the
shoulder of the survival curve at low concentrations and to increase
the slope at high concentrations. The effect on the shoulder
appears to be due to oxidation of endogenous nonprotein sulfhydryls
and reduced pyridine nucleotides (Harris and Biaglow, 1972), biochemicals that would normally effect rapid chemical repair of certain
single hit-type lesions. The slope effect, on the other hand, may
have been described for the electron-affinic compounds. In addition,
cells pretreated with Diamide and maintained at 0°C remained sensitized after the removel of Diamide. At zero degrees the metabolic
regeneration of the thiols and pyridine nucleotides was inhibited
(Harris and Power, 1973). Diamide also sensitizes in air (Fig. 9,
Chapman, 1973).

Another thiol-binding reactive agent that has been tested as
a radiosensitizer of cells is NEM (Sinclair, 1975). NEM is quite
effective at low concentrations as a sensitizer of cells under
oxygenated conditions (Sinclair, 1975). NEM, unlike Diamide, is
less specific for cellular nonprotein thiols. It reacts with both
protein and nonprotein thiols and DNA. The reaction with protein

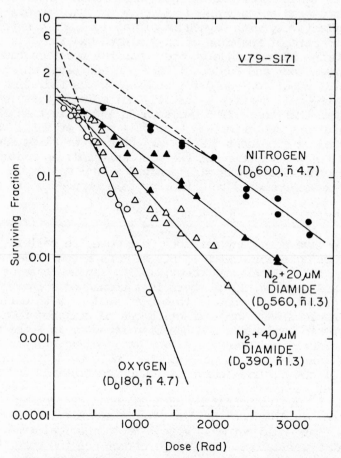

Figure 8. Effect of Diamide on the survival of V79-S171 cells
irradiated in air or nitrogen in the presence of 20
M and 40 M Diamide. The apparent OER is 3.3.
Survival curve parameters were estimated by eye; each
point is the mean of at least two experiments (Harris and
Power, 1973).

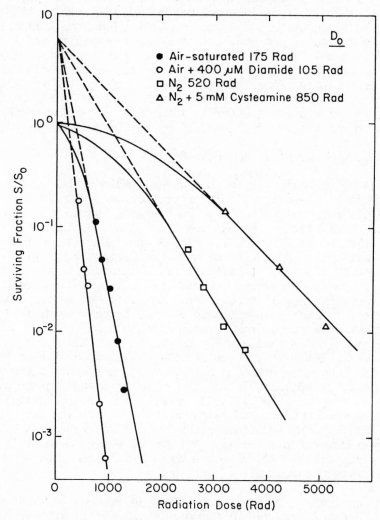

Figure 9. Survival curves for Chinese Hamster cells irradiated
under conditions exhibiting near maximum radiosensitivity and near maximum radioprotection (Chapman
et al, 1973).

thiols alters enzyme activities believed to be involved in the repair of radiation damage. It has been suggested that the primary effect of NEM on the radiation response of cells is due to the removal of a "Q" factor involved in the repair of radiation damage. Presumably, this "Q" factor is a sulfhydryl-containing enzyme (Sinclair, 1975). It is interesting to note that other workers claim to have a glutathione deficient mutant human cell line that does not show the oxygen enhancement ratio (Revesz, et al, 1979) for DNA "breaks". This cell line has the same non protein thiol content as relative to other cells. The deficiency in glutathione appears to be in the final step in biosynthesis of the tripeptide. The reported effects on DNA breakage with these cells may be due to a deficiency of glutathione for a glutathione requiring enzyme involved in the repair of the radiation damage (Revesz, et al, 1979).

RADIOPROTECTORS AND RADIATION RESPONSE

Addition of chemicals to the culture medium prior to irradiation of the cells has resulted in either protection or sensitization of the cells. In an unique publication, based in part on a long series of observations, Chapman and his colleaques demonstrated such effects (Chapman et al., 1973). Fig. 9 shows survival curves for Chinese hamster cells irradiated under conditions exhibiting near maximum and minimum radiosensitivities, obtained with the radio-sensitizer Diamide under oxic conditions and the radioprotector cysteamine under hypoxic conditions. Survival curves for cells irradiated under air-saturated and acutely hypoxic conditions have been included for comparison. These results show that the radio-sensitivity of cells made acutely hypoxic is not a minimum. The interpretation of these results led Chapman to suggest that the cellular target environment is an important component in the expression of potentially lethal free-radical damage in the cellular target(s). Chapman et al., (1973) found that dimethylsulfoxide (DMSO) protected against radiation damage by competing with cellular targets for .OH and had no effect on the radical repairing or radical-fixing species within the cell. T-butanol, while not as effective a radioprotector as DMSO, also had no effect on the environment near the target molecules.

Radioprotection by cysteamine (Fig. 9) as well as by other thiols (Chapman et al., 1973; Chapman et al., 1975) such as dithiothreitol does not appear to be the result of .OH scavenging although thiols are quite reactive with this radical (Adams and Jameson, 1977; Adams, 1979). It is believed that cysteamine protection reflects the total amount of radical damage in cellular targets which can be chemically repaired by hydrogen donating species (resulting in enhanced cell viability). The thiol protectors increase the hydrogen donating species in the target area.

Chapman's work suggests that DMSO and dithiothreitol (DTT) are

protecting cells by different mechanisms. In the case of the former
it is by scavenging the hydroxyl radical and in the case of the
later it is by providing reducing equivalents to the pool of
reducing substrates that are available within the cell to repair
radical damage. When determining the effect of a mixture of DMSO
and dithiothreitol on the radiation response it was found that
(Fig. 10) dithiothreitol and DMSO separately protected against the
damaging effects of radiation and when they were used in combination
their effects were additive. These results indicate that protection
against hydroxylradical damage was occurring and that there was a
further increase in the pool of hydrogen donating species (Biaglow
et al, 1981).

        An additional problem that arises with the use of radioprotecting
agents is the ability of these agents to consume oxygen by chemical
reaction and to stimulate cellular oxygen utilization. We have
studied both phenomena and have found that dithiothreitol is quite
potent in stimulating cellular oxygen utilization and that such
stimulation is in part dependent upon the cell cycle (Biaglow, 1982).
The stimulation of oxygen utilization by a chemical reaction with
oxygen is seen in Fig. 11. The most potent stimulator of oxygen
uptake in the medium was found to be cysteine followed by cysteamine,
dithiothreitol and glutathione. Stimulation of oxygen utilization
is in part dependent upon trace metal ions such as copper and iron
present in the growth medium and is reduced by 1/2 when catalase is
present. In metal free phosphate buffered saline, practically no
stimulation of oxygen utilization occurs. It is important to
recognize that thiol agents may in part protect via indirect
mechanisms resulting in depletion of dissolved oxygen and thereby
indirectly protecting cells against ionizing radiation (see previous
discussion) Biaglow (1981).

RADICALS AND CELL INACTIVATION

        In his careful studies, Chapman suggests that approximately
82% of the radiation inactivation (cell death) measured for air-
saturated cells is due to the fixation of target radicals (62% of
the target radicals are produced from .OH and 20% from the direct
effect) by oxygen (approximately 65%) and other endogenous electron
affinic substances (approximately 17%). The remaining 18% of
cellular inactivation or cell death may result from irrepairable or
lethal damage to cellular target(s) by direct action. Moreover,
the extent to which the indirect action of e_{aq}^{-} and H^{+} contribute
to the remaining cell inactivation is not known. There is at the
present time no comprehensive mechanism that will account for all
of the effects of ionizing radiation on mammalian cells (Alper,
1979).

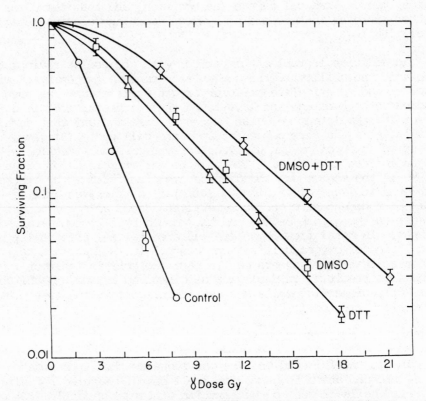

Figure 10. Survival curves for Chinese hamster V79-379 lung cells
irradiated in the presence of 1 M DMSO or 20 mM
dithiotreitol (DTT) alone or in combination.

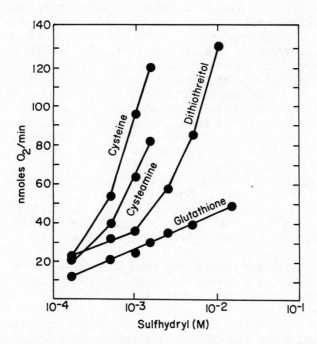

Figure 11. Oxygen consumption by different thiols when added to McCoy's 5A medium containing 10% calf serum and 0.02 M HEPES, pH 7.4.

RESPIRATORY INHIBITION AND RADIATION RESPONSE

        Inhibition of Cellular Oxygen Utilization. As indicated
previously the chief reason for hypoxic cells existing in tumors
is that the metabolic consumption of oxygen creates hypoxic cells
and results in a lowered response to ionizing radiation. Altering
the radiation response of tumors might then become concerned with
either direct inhibition of cellular oxygen utilization or some
combination of inhibition of this utilization combined with breathing
hyperbaric oxygen (Biaglow, 1981). By examing the data of Gullino
(1975) with respect to oxygen consumption of rat tumors it is
readily seen that the oxygen consumption can vary between tumors as
well as within an individual tumor (Fig. 12). Gullino's 1975 data
demonstrates the differences in diffusion distance of oxygen for
the most rapid oxygen consuming tumor compared to the least utilization. The various high and low QO_2 values for the different tumors
are seen in parenthesis to the left of the curve. From the data
seen in Fig. 12 it is possible to conclude the following:
        1.   As the tumor size increases the diffusion distance, at a
        partial pressure of 1 mm O_2, increases from 22 to 38 μm for
        the hepatocarcinoma, from 29 to 39 μm for the Walker 256 car-
        cinoma, from 30 to 100 μm for the DS tumor and from 61 to 180
        μm for the 4956 tumor.
        2.   The increase in diffusion distance is rather dramatic for
        the DS and 4956 tumors, both of which have low QO_2 values.
        3.   If the partial pressure of oxygen is increased from 1 mm
        to 160 mm there is an increase in diffusion distance which
        is a constant factor of 12.7 for all tumors.

        Gullino, 1975 and others (O_2 transport, Grote et al, 1975)
have shown that as the amount of oxygen delivered to the tumor is
increased there is not necessarily an increase in the steady state
oxygen tension. On the contrary, there is a greater utilization
(Gullino, 1975). Inhibition of oxygen utilization by those tumors
or a condition where the oxygen utilization is most likely to
increase, such as breathing hyperbaric oxygen, would produce an
increase in the diffusion distance. In Fig. 13 it is seen that as
the partial pressure of oxygen is increased for 10, 50 and 90
percent inhibition of cellular oxygen utilization, a corresponding
increase in diffusion distance appears. The greatest increases are
seen when the cellular oxygen utilization is inhibited by 90%.

CRABTREE EFFECT AND RADIATION RESPONSE

        Respiratory inhibition data indicate that oxygen sparing
mechanisms are very efficient in sensitizing hypoxic cells within
multicellular spheroids to radiation. (Biaglow, 1980). However,
many of these drugs are too toxic for use in vivo, the chemotherapy
drugs nonwithstanding (Hetzel, 1981). Other approaches have been
considered that involve the use of drugs that might release

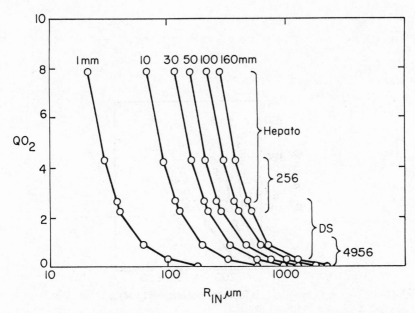

Figure 12. Increase in diffusion. Diffusion distance for different tumors with different QO_2 values obtained from Gullino, 1975. The diffusion distance was calculated from the following formula:

$$R_{in} = \sqrt{\frac{P_O}{\overline{QO}_2}} \times \mu M$$

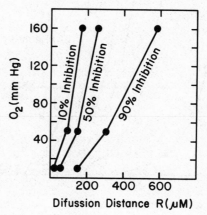

Figure 13. Increase in diffusion distance as a function of partial
          pressure of oxygen and inhibition of oxygen utilization.
          Data was taken from Tannoch and equation in Figure 12
          legend used for calculation of diffusion distances.

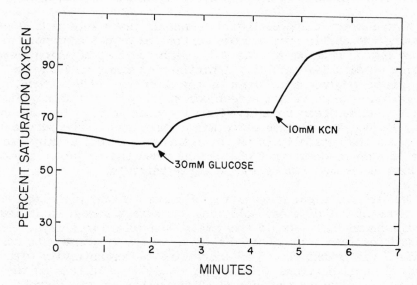

Figure 14. Increase in steady state oxygen tension caused by glucose inhibition of the oxygen utilization of Chinese hamster ovary cells. The effect of complete inhibition by cyanide addition is also seen. Data from Biaglow, 1969.

respiratory inhibitors within the tumor tissue or use of specific
physiological controls that would alter tumor metabolism so as to
produce oxygen sparing mechanisms.

When investigating cyanide release from the nitriloside
Amygdalin and its effectiveness to sensitize multicellular spheroids
to radiation it was found to be quite effective (Biaglow and Durand,
1978). However, there does not appear to be enough beta-glucosidase
within the tumor to make this drug very attractive. Notedly, one
of the nitriloside analogues is known to be hydrolysed to cyanide
and benzaldehyde by beta-glucuronidase which is known to appear in
high concentrations in tumor tissue (Biaglow and Durand, 1978).

With respect to physiological controls tests were made to
determine the ability for glucose controlled oxygen consumption to
produce oxygen sparing effects and to enhance the radiation response
(Biaglow et al., 1970, 1971). Inhibition of tumor cell oxygen
consumpiton by glucose is known as the Crabtree (1929) effect.
This is nearly a universal effect occurring with most tumor tissue
in vitro and has been recently shown to occur in vivo (Vauple and
Theus, 1975). The glucose effects are innocuous to the surrounding
tissue and the metabolic transient returns to normal within hours.
There is some evidence that glucose enhanced the radiation response
of human and animal tumors in the early thirty's.

An early clinical observation of tumor therapy with intravenous
injections of 25% dextrose solutions and x-rays seemed to indicate
that the human tumors could thereby be sensitized to x-rays. Others
reported four cases that showed a better x-ray response with dextrose.
Likewise, rat tumors showed an increasing radiosensitivity with
intraperitoneal dextrose (Biaglow et al, 1971). Increasing sensitivity was demonstrated with the Kato rabbit sarcoma when treated
with dextrose or with dextrose and cesium iodide injections followed
by irradiation. A regiment of dextrose and x-rays followed by
insulin was tried clinically and in certain cases appeared to be of
benefit. These early observations may have suggested that glucose
enhancing effect may be due to tumor cell oxygen utilization. The
Crabtree effect was discovered in the late 20's by Crabtree, 1929,
and deals with the inhibition of cellular oxygen consumption by
glucose. The Crabtree effect has been studied intensly since its
discovery. The effect is believed to be a remnant of metabolism
that has escaped control mechanisms. For example, inhibition of
oxygen utilization would be expected to cause an oxygen sparing
effect and increase in the dissolved oxygen tension. As seen in
Fig. 14 the addition of glucose in vitro produces an increase in
the steady state concentration of oxygen provided there is no
change in stirring rate. The addition of cyanide produces a complete
inhibition of oxygen utilization and a nearly complete return to
previous values without cells. Glucose controlled cellular oxygen
utilization was then tested as a means for enhancing the radiation

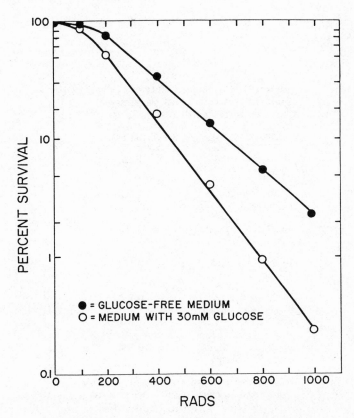

Figure 15. Radiation response for dense suspension (1×10^{6}/ml) Chinese hamster ovary cells incubated in complete growth medium in the presence and absence of glucose. Biaglow, 1969.

TABLE I

THE EFFECT OF VARIOUS CONDITIONS ON THE
RADIATION RESPONSE OF 120 HR PLATEAU
PHASE CULTURES OF V79-171B CELLS.

CONDITION	SURVIVING FRACTION
10 GY, UNSHAKEN CULTURE, 37°	0.25
10 GY, SHAKEN CULTURE, 37°	0.081
10 GY, 10^{-7}M, SHAKEN ROTENONE, 37°	0.052
10 GY, ROOM TEMP., SHAKEN, 23°	0.051
10 GY, ROOM TEMP., + ROTENONE, SHAKEN 23°	0.036
10 GY, 37° + 10^{-6}M ROTENONE, SHAKEN	0.084

THE CELLS WERE IRRADIATED UNDER THE GIVEN
CONDITIONS, REMOVED IMMEDIATELY FROM THE X-RAY
BEAM, TRYPSINIZED, COUNTED AND DILUTED TO
THE APPROPRIATE CELL DENSITY FOR CLONO-
GENIC ASSAY.

response of dense suspensions of CHO cells (Biaglow, 1969) (Fig. 15) and it can be readily seen that such suspensions show an enhanced radiation response.

Other in vitro systems have been utilized to show the effect of inhibited oxygen utilization on the radiation response. These are of course multicellular systems such as those occurring when cells are grown for prolonged periods as monolayer cultures and the cells are allowed to pile up or such systems where multicellular spheroids are allowed to be formed. The oxygen consumption and radiation response of prolonged monolayer cultures will be discussed later (Biaglow, this meeting). In monolayer systems the cells rapidly consume oxygen and produce hypoxic conditions at the bottom of the T30 flask. This is best illustrated by the experiment seen in Table 1. Cells in the culture are less sensitive to irradiation if the culture is not shaken. If the culture is shaken there is an increased response to radiation. If cellular oxygen utilization is inhibited by the respiratory inhibitor Rotenone or by lowering the temperature there is a corresponding increase in radiation response. The protection afforded the culture by making them totally hypoxic is 0.4. These experiments indicate that cellular oxygen utilization must be considered when irradiating cell suspensions (Fig. 15) as well as dense monolayer cultures and multicellular spheroids in vitro. Additional work is necessary to determine if control of cellular oxygen utilization in vivo will enhance tumor response to radiation.

ACKNOWLEDGEMENT

    This work was supported by Grant No. CA 13747 awarded by the National Cancer Institute, DHEW.

REFERENCES

1. Adams, G. E. and Jameson, D. Radiat. Envir. Biophys. 17, 95, 1980
2. Adams, G. E. Radiation Sensitizers for Hypoxic Cells: Problems and Prospects in Treatment of Radioresistant Tumors, M. Abe, K. Sakamoto and T. L. Philips, eds., Elsevier/North Holland Biomedical Press.
3. (a) Alper, T. Cellular Radiobiology, Cambridge University Press Cambridge, 1979.
   (b) Biaglow, J. E., Ferencz, N. F. and Lavik, P. Radiation Res. 623-633, 1969.
4. Biaglow, J. E. and Nygaard, O. F. Biochem. Biophys. Res. Commun. 54, 874, 1973.
5. Biaglow, J. E. Pharmacology and Therapeutics, 10, 283-299, 1980.
6. Biaglow, J. E. Radiation Research 86, 212-242, 1981.
7. Biaglow, J. E. J. Chem. Ed. 58, 144-156, 1981.

8. Brady, L., ed.   Radiation Sensitizers in Cancer Management 5, Masson Pub. Co., New York, 1980.
9. Chapman, J. D.   Rad. Res. 56, 97, 1973.
10. Chapman, J. D., Dugle, D. L., Reuvers, A. P., Gillispie, C. J. and Borsam, J.,   Radiation Res.: Biomedical, Chemical and Physical Perspectives, ed.   O. F. Nygaard, H. I. Adler and W. K. Sinclair, Academic Press, New York, 478, 1975.
11. Crabtree, H. G.   Biochemical J. 23, 536-545, 1929.
12. Elkind, M. M. and Sinclair, W. K. Current topics in Radiation Res., North Holland Publishing Co., Amsterdam 1, 165, 1965.
13. Epp, E. R., Weiss, H., Ling, C. C.   Current Topics in Radiation Res. Quarterly, 11, 201, 1976.
14. Flanders, H. P. and Moore, D.   Radiation Res. 9, 422, 1958.
15. Fowler, J. F., Adams, G. E. and Denekamp, J.   Radiosensitizers of Hypoxic Cells in Solid Tumors, Cancer Treatment Rev., 3, 2277, 1976.
16. Greenstock, C. L. and Dunlap, I.   Fast Processes in Radiation Chemistry and Biology, ed. by G. E. Adams, E. M. Fielden and B. D. Michael, M. J. Wiley and Sons, London, 247, 1975.
17. Groesch, D. S. and Hopwood, L. E.   Biological Effects of Radiation, Second Edition, Academic Press, New York, 1979.
18. Grote, J. Reneau, D. and Thews, G. V.   In Advances in Experimental Medicine and Biology, 75, Plenum Press, New York, 1975.
19. Gullino, P. M.   In Advances in Experimental Medicine and Biology, ed. by J. Grote, D. Reneau and G. Thews, 75, 521-536, 1975.
20. Hall, E. J. and Biaglow, J. E.   Int. J. Rad. Oncol. Biol. Phys. 2, 521, 1977.
21. Hall, E. J.   Radiobiology for the Radiologist, Harper, New York, 1978.
22. Harris, J. W. and Power, J. A.   Radiation Res. 56, 97, 1973.
23. Harris, J. W. and Biaglow, J. E.   Biochem. Biophys. Res. Commun. 54, 874, 1972.
24. Hetzel, F.   In Press, Cancer Clinical Trials. 1981.
25. Millar, B. C., Fielden, E. M. and Steele.   Int. J. Radiation Biol. 36, 177, 1979.
26. Painter, R. B.   Radiation Biology in Cancer Research, ed. by R. E. Meyer and H. R. Withers, Raven Press, New York, 59 1980.
27. Roots, R. and Okada, S.   Radiation Res. 64, 306, 1975.
28. Revesz, L., Edgre, M. and Larson, A., Proc. VI Int. Cong. Radiation Research, Tokyo, ed. by S. Okada, M. Imamura, T. Terashima and H. Yamaguchi, Toppan Printing Co., Ltd. Tokyo, Japan, 1979.
29. Sinclair, W. K.   Radiation Research, Biomedical Chemical and Physical Perspectives.   Academic Press, New York, 1975.
30. Ward, J.   Adv. Radiation Biol. 5, 181, 1977.
31. Watts, M. E., Whillans, D. W. and Adams, Ge. E.   Int. J. Radiat. Biol 27, 259, 1975.

32. Vaupel, P. and Thews, G.   In Advances in Experimental Medicine
        and Biology, Ed. by J. Grote, D. Reneau and G. Thews,
        <u>75</u>, 547 553, 1975.

DIFFERENTIAL RESPONSE TO HEAT OF METASTATIC AND NON-METASTATIC RAT

MAMMARY TUMORS

Milton B. Yatvin, John Vorpahl, Untae Kim

University of Wisconsin, Department of Human Oncology,
WCCC, Madison, WI 53792; Roswell Park Memorial Institute,
Department of Pathology, Buffalo, NY 14263

INTRODUCTION

Interest in the use of heat for cancer treatment has increased markedly in recent years (1-4). Information has accumulated that such hyperthermia causes a selective and irreversible inhibition of metabolism in certain animal and human tumors correlated to cell killing (5-8). It remains uncertain, however, whether and under which conditions heat exerts a specific influence on tumor tissue since much of the information available is based on cells cultured in vitro. Nevertheless, the potential application of hyperthermia in the treatment of cancer is extremely attractive since, with the exception of systemic chemotherapy, which is a notoriously blunt weapon, regional and whole body hyperthermia are the only treatment modalities presently available which could address the major problem of human cancer: the metastatic lesion. It is not known, however, whether metastasizing tumors are more susceptible to hyperthermic treatment than non-metastasizing ones, although in vitro studies are consistent with this possibility (9). The metastatic capacities of a tumor cell are related to its surface (10,11) and one of the major mechanisms of action of hyperthermia is thought to act via the membrane (12,13). It, therefore, was of interest to compare the membrane properties and heat sensitivity in two closely related tumor strains of which one metastasizes whereas the other does not.

METHODS

The pair of tumors utilized is the metastasizing SMT-2A mammary adenocarcinoma and its non-metastasizing counterpart MT-W9B.

The tumors are implanted in the right inner femoral area of W/Fu rats by injecting o.2 ml of a 10% cell suspension. Tumor size is measured by caliper, and treatment is carried out when the tumors have attained a size of 5x5 mm, i.e. about 4-5 weeks after implantation. The tumor SMT-2A had already formed metastases a few days after implantation. Hyperthermic treatment is carried out by immersing the tumor-bearing leg of the rat anesthetized with chloral hydrate into a water bath. The water bath is covered with floating polyethylene spheres to insulate and reduce evaporation and is continuously monitored by means of an electronic thermometer and adjusted by a Tecam T40 controller. Most heat treatments are carried out at 43.5°C for 60 minutes.

Following treatment, tumor size is measured daily, and the results are expressed as percentage of animals which do not resume tumor growth at a given day. The measure of tumor growth is its volume index (TVI) and is calculated from the measurement of the minor axis (W) and the major axis (L) of the tumor according to the following formula: $TVI = (W)^2 \times L$. Proteins are determined from a homogenate prepared of tumor cells. Lipids are then extracted with chloroform/methanol according to Bligh and Dyer (14). Phosphorus content is determined, and fatty acids are obtained by transesterification of the extract with methanolic HCl under reflux at 70°C for 2 hours. The fatty acid esters are separated by gas chromatography on a 10% DEGS column using an appropriate temperature gradient program. Peaks are identified by comparison with authentic standards and are quantified with a Hewlett Packard integrator.

Results

The percentage of non-metastasizing MT-W9B mammary adenomas displaying no regrowth as a function of the time after different hyperthermic treatment is show in figure 1. Delay of tumor growth by heat treatment is short, and after 5 days almost all tumors have regrown. Moreover, no significant difference between the behavior after the various treatment schedules is discernible. On the contrary, growth of the metastasizing tumor SMT-2A is markedly retarded following hyperthermic treatment at 43.5°C for 60 minutes, but is much less so after a shorter treatment time or at a lower temperature (Figure 2). The difference is clearly apparent when the behavior of both tumors following heating to 43.5°C for 60 minutes is shown on the same scale (Figure 3) and is also discernible from the tumor volume index (not shown).

The two mammary adenocarcinomas also are clearly distinct with respect to their fatty acid composition (Table 1 and 2). About twice as much arachidonic acid is present in the non-metastasizing compared to the metastasizing tumor. On the other hand, the metastasizing tumor contains less linoleic acid and displays a higher ratio of palmitic to stearic acid than the non-metastasizing

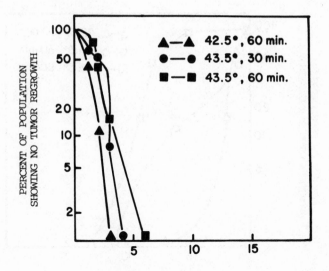

TIME AFTER TREATMENT (DAYS)

Figure 1. Plot of the percent of the population showing no tumor
regrowth of MT-W9B against time after treatment. Tumors
were grown in legs of female Wistar Furth rats weighing
200 gms. When the tumors reached a size of 5x5 mm
(4-5 weeks), the animals were anesthetized and the tumor
bearing leg heated in a water bath.

one. The ratio of proteins to phospholipids in metastasizing tumors
is also less than one-half that of non-metastasizing tumors.

Discussion

The two rat adenocarcinomas utilized have been described in
detail (10). The metastasizing SMT-2A tumor displays infiltrative
growth and metastasizes along the lymphatic route into lung, liver,
and bone within a few days after implantation. The non-metastasizing
MT-W9B adenocarcinoma remains restricted to the site of implantation
and grows by expansion. The non-metastasizing tumor is immunogenic
whereas the metastasizing tumor is not. Membrane marker enzymes
such as glycosyltransferases and 5'-nucleotidase display higher
levels in metastasizing tumors and may appear in serum. Thus, it
appears that a characteristic feature of metastasizing tumors is

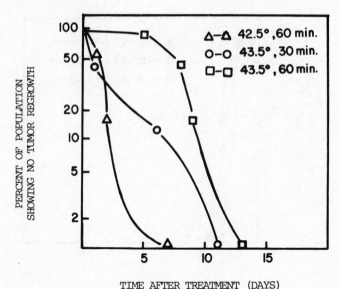

Figure 2. Same experimental procedure as Figure 1 except for the SMT-2A tumor.

its extremely unstable plasma membrane structure from which incompletely assembled constituents are continuously shed (10). Such a shedding may weaken and destroy the bonds between cells and clear a path for the dispersion of tumor cells. The present finding that metastasizing tumors have lower levels of arachidonic acid may be seen as a response to plasma membrane instability which in conjunction with the increased linoleic acid content and the decreased ratio palmitic to stearic acid may reflect an attempt by the cell to cope with the loss of membrane material. A preferential shedding of protein constituents is evident also from the observed lower ratio of protein to phospholipid in metastasizing compared to non-metastasizing tumors. One may postulate that the tumor cell attempts to increase the microviscosity of the membrane by reducing its content of arachidonic acid. Such "homeoviscous adaptation" has been observed in several instances (15) and, in the SMT-2A may be needed to compensate for the loss of proteins from the membrane. Preliminary studies using fluorescence polarization to assess the microviscosity of these tumor cells, however, have not indicated large differences so that the relatively greater amount of longer chain saturated fatty acids and the decrease in arachidonic acid

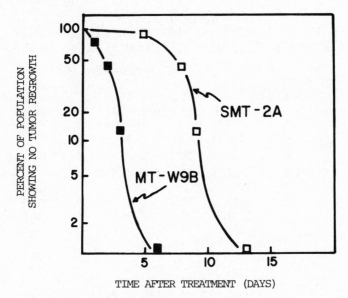

Figure 3.   Same experimental procedure as Figure 1 but combines the
            MT-W9B and the SMT-2A tumor data.

may have compensated for the loss of proteins. The alterations in
the membrane, however, could still be of such nature that its
reserve capacity to maintain its integrity in response to a hyperthermic insult is compromised (16). Indeed, whereas the correlation
between microviscosity, lipid composition and thermal sensitivity
is quite good in prokaryotic cells, deviations are sometimes observed in eukaryotic cells due to the greater complexity involved
in maintaining homeoviscous regulation (17). Nevertheless, such a
correlation has been demonstrated in ascites cells (18). When these
cells are made more fluid by addition of unsaturated fatty acids
to diets of host mice, their sensitivity to heat is increased (19).
Our present biochemical analyses on tumor cells were carried out
on whole cell homogenate, and more detailed information on composition, enzymatic endowment and biosynthesis of isolated tumor
membranes will be obtained from studies in progress.

     The greater heat sensitivity of the metastasizing tumor com-
pared to the non-metastasizing one is of great interest. Aside
from the potential implications for cancer therapy, which obviously
must await confirmation on a much larger spectrum of metastasizing
and non-metastasizing tumors, this observation also seems to

TABLE 1
FATTY ACID COMPOSITION AND PROTEIN PHOSPHOLIPID RATIO
IN THE NON-METASTASIZING MT-W9B MAMMARY ADENOCARCINOMA

TUMOR VOLUME (W^2L)	PROTEIN PHOSPHOLIPID	GAS CHROMATOGRAPHY - AREA %					
		16:0	16:1	18:0	18:1	18:2	20:4
514	6.06	23.77	4.41	14.06	27.36	9.56	20.83
650	7.69	25.23	5.42	14.08	27.20	7.86	20.21
456	5.85	24.65	5.78	13.76	28.88	9.61	17.31
627	8.40	22.78	5.16	14.78	24.31	8.79	24.19
562±92	7.00±1.25	24.11 ±1.07	5.19 ±0.58	14.17 ±0.43	26.94 ±1.91	8.96 ±0.82	20.63 ±2.82

TABLE 2
FATTY ACID COMPOSITION AND PROTEIN PHOSPHOLIPID RATIO
IN THE METASTASIZING SMT-2A MAMMARY ADENOCARCINOMA

TUMOR VOLUME (W^2L)	PROTEIN PHOSPHOLIPID	GAS CHROMATOGRAPHY - AREA %					
		16:0	16:1	18:0	18:1	18:2	20:4
150	2.04	22.38	4.11	19.91	29.53	12.40	11.66
331	3.66	20.43	4.32	19.31	30.86	14.54	10.55
247	5.00	20.09	4.86	15.41	31.86	19.71	8.06
343	2.79	19.20	3.57	17.21	34.47	15.81	9.74
469	2.96	19.06	6.15	20.40	30.77	12.31	11.31
308±119	3.29±1.07	20.23 ±1.33	4.60 ±0.98	18.45 ±2.09	31.50 ±1.86	14.95 ±3.05	10.26 ±1.44

establish another link between alterations in the membrane and
sensitivity to heat. Nevertheless, other explanations for the
greater heat sensitivity of the metastatic tumor are conceivable
and must be tested in the future. Thus, blood flow in the metastasizing tumor was found to be only about one-half of that in the
non-metastasizing tumor (20), and the greater response to hyperthermia of the metastasizing tumor might be explained on the basis
of a smaller heat transfer from the tumor. Whatever the reasons
may be for the differences in sensitivity to hyperthermic treatment
between metastasizing and non-metastasizing tumors, they seem to
open potentially valuable avenues of approach for the understanding
of mechanisms of metastatic behavior and for the treatment of
metastatic lesions.

Summary

Metastasizing and non-metastasizing transplantable mammary tumors were implanted into female W/Fu rats. A pair of tumors were employed, the SMT-2A and MT-W9B. When these tumors were exposed to water bath heating at 43.5°C for 60 minutes, a significantly longer tumor-free growth delay was obtained in the metastasizing tumor compared to its non-metastasizing counterpart. The protein to phospholipid ratio and the content of arachidonic acid was lower in the metastasizing tumor than in the non-metastasizing one. By way of apparent compensation, the metastasizing tumor contained more linoleic and stearic acid. These observations suggest a relation between metastasizing capacity, thermal sensitivity, and membrane composition.

Acknowledgements

We are grateful to Dr. George Gerber for his interest in these studies and advice and help during the preparation of this manuscript. These studies were supported in part by NCI Grant 5P01 CA 19278 and Grant CA 24215.

References

1. Cavaliere, R., Ciocatto, E. C., Giovanella, B. C., Heidelberger, C., Johnson, R. O., Margottini, M., Mondovi, B., Moricca, G., and Rossi-fanelli, A. Selective Heat Sensitivity of Cancer Cells. Cancer 20:1351-1381, 1967.
2. Stehlin, J. S. Hyperthermic Profusion with Chemotherapy for Cancer of the Extremities. Surgical Gynecology Obstetrics 128:305-318, 1969.
3. Pettigrew, R. T., Galt, J. N., Ludgate, C. M., Smith, A. N. Clinical Affects of Whole Body Hyperthermia in Advanced Malignancy. British Journal of Medicine 4:679-682, 1974.
4. Streffer, C. Cancer Therapy by Hyperthermia and Radiation, Urban and Schwarzenberg, Munich, Baltimore, pgs. 3-341, 1978.
5. Dickson, J. A. The Effects of Hyperthermia on Animal Tumor Systems, In: Selective Heat Sensitivity of Cancer Cells, eds., Rossi-fanelli, A., Cavaliere, R., Mondovi, B., Moricca, G., Recent Results in Cancer Research 59:43-111, 1977.
6. Giovanella, B. C., Stehlin, J. S., Morgan, A. C. Selective Lethal Effect of Supra-normal Temperature in Human Neoplastic Cells, Cancer Research 36:3944-3950, 1976.
7. Overgaard, K., Overgaard, J. Investigations on a Possibility of a Thermic Tumor Therapy. I. Short-wave Treatment of a Transplanted Isologous Mouse Mammary Carcinoma, European Journal of Cancer 8:65-78, 1972.

8. Crile, G. The Effects of Heat and Radiation on Cancers Implanted in the Feet of Mice, Cancer Research 23:372-380, 1963.
9. Tomasovic, S. P., and Nicolson, G. L. Heterogeneity in Hyperthermic Killing of Mammary Tumor Cell Clones of Differing Metastatic Potential, Abs. DG-14, 29th Annual Meeting of the Radiation Research Society, June 1981.
10. Kim, U. Factors Influencing Metastasis of Breast Cancer, McGuire, W. L., ed., Breast Cancer, Vol. 3, Plenum Publishing Corp., 1979, pgs. 1-49.
11. Martines-Polomo, A. The Nature of Neoplastic Cell Membranes, Experimental and Molecular Pathology 31:219-235, 1979.
12. Yatvin, M. B. The Influence of Membrane Lipid Composition and Procaine on Hyperthermic Death of Cells, Int. J. of Rad. Biol. 32:513-521, 1977.
13. Mulcahy, R. T., Gould, M. N., Hidvegi, E. G., Elson, C. E., and Yatvin, M. B. Hyperthermia and Surface Morphology of P388 Ascites Tumor Cells: Effects of Membrane Modificaions, Int. J. of Radiat. Biol. 39:95-106, 1981.
14. Bligh, E. G., and Dyer, W. J. A Rapid Method of Total Lipid Extraction and Purification. Can. J. Biochem. Physiol. 37:911-917, 1959.
15. Sinensky, C. Homeoviscous Adaptation: A Homeostatic Process that Regulates the Viscosity of Membrane Lipids in Escherichia coli. Proc. Natl. Acad. Sci. 71:522-525, 1974.
16. Helmkamp, G. M. Effects of Phospholipid Fatty Acid Composition and Membrane Fluidity on the Activity of Bovine Brain Phospholipid Exchange Position. Biochemistry 19:2050-2051, 1980.
17. Lepock, J. R., Mossicotte-Nolan, P., Rule, G. S., and Kruuv, J. Lack of a Correlation between Hyperthermic Cell Killing, Thermotolerance, and Membrane Lipid Fluidity, Radiation Research 87:300-313, 1981.
18. Harms-Ringdahl, M. Effects of the Fatty Acid Composition of Membranes on Radiosensitivity and Hyperthermia in Mice and E. Ascites Cells. Abs. #24, 2nd WCCC International Workshop on Experimental Oncology, Madison, WI, May, 1981.
19. Hidvegi, E. G., Yatvin, M. B., Dennis, W. H., and Hidveg, Eva. Effect of Altered Membrane Lipid Composition and Procaine on Hyperthermic Killing of Ascites Tumor Cells, Oncology 37:360-363, 1980.
20. Jirtle, R. L.   Blood Flow to Lymphatic Metastases in Conscious Rats. European J. of Cancer 17(1):53-60, 1981.

COMPUTER MODELING OF TUMOR HYPERTHERMIA

(A DYNAMIC LUMPED PARAMETER MODEL)

Nathan Busch, Duane F. Bruley, and Haim I. Bicher

Biomedical Engineering Department, Louisiana Tech
University, Ruston, Louisiana, 71270 and Western Tumor
Medical Group and Valley Cancer Institute, 5522 Sepulveda
Van Nuys, California, 91411

ABSTRACT

The thermal behavior of normal and neoplastic tissue is
modeled by a set of coupled ordinary differential equations. The
equations lump the tissue and tumor into individual compartments,
so that the equations are time dependent. These equations represent
an initial step in the development of a comprehensive model which
may be used in studying the dynamics and control of the system under
normo-and hyperthermic conditions.

INTRODUCTION

The treatment of solid tumors by hyperthermia and ionizing
radiation has received a growing amount of attention in recent years.
Short and Turner (4) presented an extensive work on the subject.
Other works discussing the behavior of neoplastic and normal tissue
under hyperthermic conditions include Field, et. al. (2), Nemoto
(3), and Sein and Jain (5). The most complete lumped parameter
model of a tumor-tissue system is given by Sien and Jain (4). Their
model was for a Waler 256 Carcinoma implanted in a Sprague-Dawley
rat. However, their treatment was primarily for whole body or
localized thermal treatment. The model introduced in this study
utilizes microwave radiation as the source of heat. This model is
directly applicable when radiowave frequency radiation is used.

A dynamic model of the tumor-tissue system was developed
and solved on a digital computer. The model included terms for
pulsing blood flow and levels of radiation. It is felt that the
ability to pusle the level of radiation is necessary since in
clinical application, the radiation is switched on and off to record

185

the tumor temperature. This problem may be circumvented by using
the photoilluminscent devices as discussed by Taylor (6). The
pulsitile microwave radiation may have a significantly different
effect on the system than constant radiation will. This phenomena
will occur whenever there is a natural resonance frequency occurring
in the system. The model is straight forward and is simplistic
enough to allow for initial parametric studies. These studies will
indicate which terms are important enough to be included in more
comprehensive and complex models of the tumor-tissue system.

THEORY

The first term on the right of the tumor energy balance
accounts for the convection of energy into and out of the system
by the blood. The exiting blood temperature may be assumed to be
the same as the tumor temperature. The second term on the right
accounts for the energy deposition in the tumor by the microwave
radiation. The last term on the right accounts for the transfer
of energy from the tumor to the tissue. h is the effective convective
conductance for the transport of energy between the tumor and the
tissue. The rate of heat transfer is dependent on this parameter
and its value must be determined by experimental measurements.

The lumped parameter model equations for the system
are as follows:

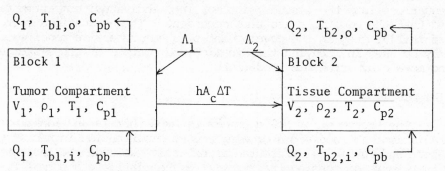

The tumor thermal energy conservation equation is

$$\frac{dT_1^*}{dt^*} = \frac{\rho_b Q_1 C_{pb} t^o (T_{b1,i}^* - T_{b1,o}^*)}{\rho_1 C_{p1}} + \frac{\Lambda_1 t^o}{\rho_1 C_{p1} (T_{max} - T^o)} - \frac{h A_s t^o (T_1^* - T_2^*)}{\rho_1 V_1 C_{p1}}$$

The tissue thermal energy conservation equation is

$$\frac{dT_2^*}{dt^*} = \frac{\rho_b Q_2 C_{pb} t^o (T_{b2,i}^* - T_{b2,o}^*)}{\rho_2 C_{p2}} + \frac{\Lambda_2 t^o}{\rho_2 C_{p2}(T_{max} - T^o)} + \frac{hA_s t^o (T_1^* - T_2^*)}{\rho_2 V_2 C_{p2}}$$

This equation is identical, in form, to the energy conservation equation for the tumor. These equations are developed such that the blood flow rate and energy deposition by the microwaves may be different for the tumor and tissue compartments. This provision allows for a more realistic simulation of the system.

These equations must be solved numerically since the physical parameters used in them are temperature dependent. This makes them nonlinear. The convective conductance "h" may be found by matching experimentally measured temperatures with the computed temperatures. The technique for accomplishing this has been discussed by Busch et al. (1).

DISCUSSION

The model described above is an initial step in the development of a complex and comprehensive model of a tumor-tissue system. Its simplicity and flexibility provides a useful tool in performing parametric, dynamic, and control studies of the physical system. The parametric studies indicate which parameters and terms need to be included in more complex models, as well as which parameters need to be measured more accurately and included in the model. The dynamic studies indicate what effect the pulsitile microwave radiation treatment will have on the temperature history of the system. The control studies will allow for the development of optimal fraction-ation schedules. The control studies will also allow for the development of automatic treatment without using invasive temper-ature measuring devices. Thus, it is clear that initial models such as the one given here may prove to be useful in the development of complex models as well as in the clinical treatment of tumors.

CONCLUSIONS

A mathematical model of the tumor-tissue system has been developed. The model is an initial step in the development of more complex and comprehensive models of the system. The model is a valuable tool in performing parametric, dynamic, and control studies.

NOMENCLATURE

A_s Surface area of the tumor, $= 4\pi r_1^2$, (cm^2)

C_{pb} Specific heat of the blood $= 0.87$ cal/gm-blood/^{o}C.

C_{pl} Specific heat of the tumor $= 0.75$ cal/gm-tumor/^{o}C.

C_{p2} Specific heat of the tissue $= 0.86$ cal/gm-tissue/^{o}C.

h Convective conductance between the tumor and tissue $=$ 1.3563×10^{-4} cal/cm^2/sec/^{o}C.

Q_1 Volumetric blood flow rate through the tumor, $(cm^3$-blood/ cm^3-tumor/sec).

Q_2 Volumetric blood flow rate through the tissue $(cm/^3$-blood/ cm^3-tissue/sec).

$T^*_{b1,i}$ Dimensionless inlet blood temperature to the tumor $= 0.0$.

$T^*_{b2,i}$ Dimensionless inlet blood temperature to the tissue $= 0.0$.

$T^*_{b1,o}$ Dimensionless exit blood temperature from the tumor $= T^*_1$.

$T^*_{b2,o}$ Dimensionless exit blood temperature from the tissue $= T^*_2$.

T^*_1 Dimensionless tumor temperature.

T^*_2 Dimensionless tissue temperature.

T_{max} Maximum hyperthermic temperature $= 45.0^o$C.

T^o Normal body temperature $= 37.0^o$C.

t^o Fundamental unit of time $= 60.0$ sec.

t^* Dimensionless time.

r_1 Tumor radius $= 1.1$ cm.

r_2 Tissue outer radius, $= 1.5$ cm.

V_1 Tumor volume $= 4/3 \pi r_1^3$.

V_2 Tissue volume $= 4/3 \pi (r_2^3 - r_1^3)$.

ρ_1 Tumor density $= 0.98$ gm-tumor/cm^3-tumor.

ρ_2 Tissue density $= 0.99$ gm-tissue/cm^3-tissue.

ρ_b Blood denisty = 1.0 gm-blood/cm^3-blood.

Λ_1 Level of radiation to the tumor = 0.035 cal/cm^3-tumor/sec.

Λ_2 Level of radiation to the tissue = 0.038 cal/cm^3-tissue/sec.

REFERENCES

1. Busch, N., D. Bruley, and H. Bicher, "Identification of Viable
   Regions in "in vitro" Spheroidal Tumors: A Mathematical
   Investigation," This publication.
2. Field, S. B., and N. M. Bleehen, "Hyperthermia in the Treatment
   of Cancer," Cancer Treatment Reviews, volume 6, 63-94,
   1979.
3. Nemoto, E. M., and H. M. Frankel, "Cerebral Oxygenation and
   Metabolism during Progressive Hyperthermia," American
   Journal of Physiology, Volume 219, Number 6, 1784-1788,
   1970.
4. Short, J. G. and P. F. Turner, "Physical Htperthermia and
   Cancer Therapy," IEEE Proceedings, Volume 68, Number 1,
   133-141, 1980.
5. Sien, H. P. and R. K. Jain, "Temperature Distribution in Normal
   and Neoplastic Tissues During Hyperthermia: Lumpted
   Parameter Analysis," Thermal Biology, Volume, 1, 1-7, 1979.
6. Taylor, L. S., "Implantable Radiators for Cancer Therapy by
   Microwave Hyperthermia," IEEE Proceedings, Volume 68,
   Number 1, 142-149, 1980.